The Use and Misuse of
Sleeping Pills

—— *A Clinical Guide* ——

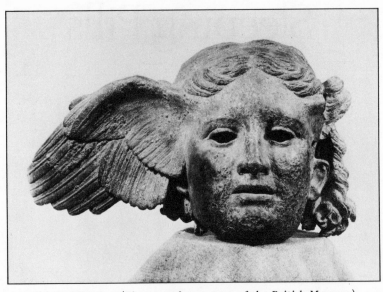

Head of Hypnos (*Photograph courtesy of the British Museum*)

The Use and Misuse of
Sleeping Pills
——A Clinical Guide——

Wallace B. Mendelson, M.D.
National Institute of Mental Health
Bethesda, Maryland

Plenum Medical Book Company
New York and London

Library of Congress Cataloging in Publication Data

Mendelson, Wallace B
  The use and misuse of sleeping pills.

  Includes bibliographical references and index.
  1. Hypnotics. 2. Insomnia — Chemotherapy. 3. Medication abuse. I. Title.
[DNLM: 1. Hypnotics and sedatives — Pharmacodynamics. 2. Hypnotics and sedatives — Adverse effects. 3. Insomnia — Drug therapy. QV85 M537u]
RM325.M46   615'.782   79-21856
ISBN 0-306-40370-6

Preface

Hypnos (the Greek god of sleep) and Thanatos (death) were the twin sons of Nyx, the goddess of night (Fox, 1964). Hypnos lived in a dusky valley in the land of the Cimerians, watered by Lethe, the river of forgetfulness. He brought sleep to both men and gods, and sometimes sent his sons Morpheus, Icelus, and Phantasus to appear in dreams. At the door of his abode grew poppies and other herbs which induce sleep (Hamilton, 1961). This book deals with these herbs and their subsequent imitations.

Before launching into an examination of hypnotics, it might be well to comment briefly on the manner in which this was written, and to acknowledge the help of a number of individuals. My intention was that this be useful not only for the physician or scientist, but also for the student. Thus each chapter contains an introductory section which provides background material. Chapter 3, for instance, describes the general principles of drug absorption, distribution, and metabolism before discussing the pharmacologic properties of each hypnotic. In addition, each chapter concludes with a section which summarizes the main issues.

This book was made possible by the continued encouragement and many helpful suggestions of Dr. Richard Jed Wyatt and Dr. J. Christian Gillin. Dr. William E. Bunney has been supportive throughout the course of this work. A number of persons were kind enough to comment on various chapters, for which thanks go to Drs. William C. Dement, David C. Kay, Daniel F. Kripke, William Potter, Seymour Perlin, Laurence S. Jacobs, Donald W. Goodwin, and Johanna S. R. Mendelson. My interest in this area was stimulated by working with the Institute of Medicine on a study of insomnia and hypnotics, for which I am grateful to Dr. David A.

Hamburg and the Institute staff. Miss Susan Dawson very kindly assisted in the preparation of the manuscript.

Lastly, this book has been written by me as a private individual. The views expressed do not necessarily reflect those of the Public Health Service, the National Institute of Mental Health, or the Institute of Medicine.

WALLACE B. MENDELSON

Bethesda, Maryland

Contents

1 Basic Concepts about Sleep and Insomnia 1

History 1
The Sleep Stages 3
   Waking 3
   NonREM Sleep 4
      Stage 1 4
      Stage 2 4
      Stages 3 and 4 5
   REM Sleep 6
Influences on the Appearance of Sleep Stages 7
Physiologic Regulation of Sleep 9
   Passive versus Active Model 9
   The Neurotransmitters 10
   Circulating Humors 12
Hypnotics and Sleep Regulation 12
Sleep Deprivation 13
The Need for Sleep 15
Insomnia 16
Summary and Conclusions 23

2 The Prevalence of Sleep Disturbance and Hypnotic Use 25

Surveys of Reported Sleep Disturbance 25
Types of Sleep Complaints 30

Surveys of Hypnotic Use 31
Patient–Physician Interaction 33
Prescriptions for Outpatients 35
Prescribing Hypnotics in Hospital Practice 36
Summary and Conclusions.................................... 36

3   Pharmacology of Prescription Hypnotics 39

Pharmacologic Considerations 40
Barbiturates 45
    History 45
    Actions 47
    Structure and Classification 47
    Alterations in Metabolism and Excretion: Illness, Old Age,
        Enzyme Induction 50
    Chronic Administration 51
Benzodiazepines 52
    History 52
    Flurazepam 53
    Nitrazepam 55
    Temazepam 55
    Other Properties of Benzodiazepines 55
Nonbarbiturate, Nonbenzodiazepine Hypnotics 56
    Chloral Hydrate and Derivatives 56
    Methaqualone 58
    Piperidinedione Derivatives........................... 59
        Glutethimide...................................... 59
        Methyprylon 60
    Ethchlorvynol 60
    Ethinamate... 61
Summary and Conclusions.................................... 61

4   The Efficacy of Hypnotics 63

Methodologic Considerations................................ 64
    Possible Measures of Efficacy 64
    Subject Selection 65
    Other Methodological Issues 66
Efficacy Studies in Specific Disorders 67

Reference Section: Efficacy Studies in Normal Volunteers
    and "Insomniacs" 69
  Barbiturates 70
  Benzodiazepines 72
    Flurazepam 72
    Nitrazepam 76
    Temazepam 77
  Nonbarbiturate, Nonbenzodiazepine Hypnotics 78
    Chloral Hydrate 78
    Methaqualone 79
    Glutethimide 81
    Methyprylon 82
    Ethchlorvynol 83
  Summary and Conclusions 83

5 Suicide and Hypnotics 85

Incidence 85
Traits of the Victim 89
Clinical Toxicity 92
  Barbiturates 92
  Benzodiazepines 93
  Nonbarbiturate, Nonbenzodiazepine Hypnotics 93
    Chloral Hydrate 93
    Methaqualone 94
    Glutethimide 95
    Ethchlorvynol 95
Treatment 96
Prevention 98
Summary and Conclusions 99

6 Residual Daytime Effects of Hypnotics 101

Electrophysiologic Residual Effects 101
Psychomotor Measures of Residual Effects 104
Subjective Evaluation of Daytime Performance 111
Hypnotics and Driving 112
Summary and Conclusions 113

7 Interactions with Ethanol 115

General Considerations 116
Barbiturates 116
Benzodiazepines 118
Nonbarbiturate, Nonbenzodiazepine Hypnotics 122
    Chloral Hydrate 122
    Methaqualone 123
    Glutethimide 123
Summary and Conclusions.................................... 125

8 Hypnotic Dependence 127

Classical Drug Abuse 128
Dependence in Medical Practice 129
    Dependence on Extremely Large Doses 129
    Prolonged Use of Recommended Doses 130
        Incidence and Contributing Factors 130
        Drug Qualities Related to Prolonged Use 133
Summary and Conclusions.................................... 138

9 Hypnotics and the Elderly 141

Pharmacology in the Elderly 142
Efficacy Studies 145
Toxicity 150
Summary and Conclusions.................................... 151

10 Other Pharmacologic Approaches 153

Over-the-Counter Hypnotics 153
    Compounds Used in OTC Hypnotics 154
        Methapyrilene.................................... 154
        Scopolamine 155
        Bromides 156
    Efficacy 156
    Federal Regulation 157

L-Tryptophan 159
Ethanol 160
Summary and Conclusions.................................. 161

11   Nonpharmacologic Treatment of Insomnia 163

Counseling and Psychotherapy 163
Behavioral Therapies 164
   General Considerations 164
   Relaxation Procedures 166
   Conditioning-Derived Therapies 169
   Attributional Therapy 171
   Behavioral Self-Management.............................. 173
Summary and Conclusions.................................. 173

12   Conclusion: Implications for Medical Practice 177

Summary 177
Approach to the Insomniac Patient 182
   Evaluation 182
   The Decision Whether to Give Hypnotics 183
      Acute or Intermittent Insomnia............................ 184
      Chronic Insomnia 184
   When Hypnotics Are Prescribed 184

References 187

Index 217

CHAPTER 1

Basic Concepts about Sleep and Insomnia

HISTORY

In the 1870s, the English physician Richard Caton described spontaneous electrical activity in the brains of animals. The observation of these "feeble currents of the brain" was all the more remarkable in that it was done without the benefit of electronic amplification, which was not available for biological research for another 50 years (Brazier, 1973). Caton went on to observe that these electrical events could be altered by sensory stimulation, anaesthesia, and sleep (Schoenberg, 1974). It was not until 1929 that Hans Berger, a German psychiatrist, recorded similar phenomena from electrodes placed on the scalp of humans. Over the next 10 years, he reported that these recordings, which he referred to as *electroencephalograms*, changed with age and sensory stimulation, and were abnormal during epileptic seizures. Eight years after Berger's original observations, Loomis, Harvey, and Hobart (1937) studied the first electroencephalographic recordings during human sleep. They reported that sleep is composed of several discontinuous stages, and speculated that their spontaneous changes were governed by "internal stimuli." Although the descriptions have evolved over the years, the observation that sleep is composed of several recurring electrophysiologic stages remains an important principle in sleep research.

While these important electrophysiologic observations were being reported, a number of writers were also making remarkably prophetic speculations about another important aspect of sleep—dreaming. The

1

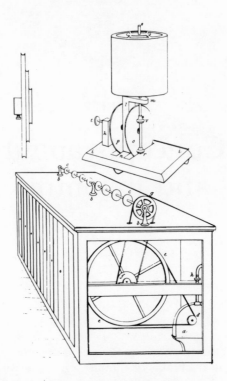

FIGURE 1. Water-powered recorder built by Richard Caton (Caton, 1887).

psychiatrist Griesinger (1868) and later several others believed that the eyes moved during dreaming. In 1895 Freud observed that the major muscles of the body relax when one dreams. MacWilliam (1923) distinguished between "undisturbed" and "disturbed" sleep; in the latter (in which he thought dreaming might take place), there were increased blood pressure and pulse, and changes in the rate of respiration.

The electrophysiologic studies and the speculations on the physiology of dreaming came together with the studies of Aserinsky and Kleitman at the University of Chicago in 1953. They discovered that during human sleep there were periods characterized by rapid conjugate eye movements, during which the EEG displayed an activated pattern of low-amplitude waves predominantly of 15–20 and 5–8 cycles per second (cps). During these periods, which came to be known as Rapid Eye Movement (REM) sleep, there was an increase in the rate of the heartbeat and respiration. Perhaps the most exciting finding was that when Aserinsky and Kleitman aroused persons from REM sleep, about three-fourths of them reported that they had been dreaming, and a few more reported "the feeling of having dreamed." When they awakened subjects from sleep which did not contain REMs (nonREM sleep), about 9% reported dreaming and a similar number reported a sensation of having been dreaming.

During the next decade REM sleep was characterized more fully. Jouvet and Michel (1959) observed that muscle tone decreased markedly in the REM sleep of animals, and Ralph Berger reported a similar finding in humans in 1961. Dement and Kleitman (1957) found that REM sleep occurred in the cyclic fashion throughout the night, roughly every 90–100 min. They classified sleep into REM sleep and four stages of nonREM sleep, an approach which with some revisions (Rechtschaffen & Kales, 1968) continues to be widely employed. Authors including Oswald (1962) and Jouvet (1962) began to stress that sleep was not a unitary process; in fact, many physiologic measures suggested that REM was as different from nonREM sleep as the latter was from waking. Hence, REM sleep, nonREM sleep, and waking come to be known as the three *states of consciousness*.

THE SLEEP STAGES

The sleep stages are commonly studied by examining three basic physiologic measures: (1) the electroencephalogram (EEG), derived from an electrode attached to the scalp (what is actually recorded is usually the difference in the voltage detected from an electrode on the scalp and that from a relatively neutral location such as the mastoid bone); (2) the electrooculogram (EOG), a measure of lateral movements of the eyes; and (3) the electromyogram (EMG), a measure of muscle tension obtained by taping electrodes in the area of the muscles under the chin. These three types of information are recorded on a continually moving strip of paper and are interpreted by a reader who determines the sleep stage for every sequential "epoch" (usually 30 sec). The characteristics of the sleep stages have been described in detail in Rechtschaffen and Kales (1968) and may be summarized as follows:

Waking

In a relaxed subject whose eyes are closed, the EEG shows a predominant alpha (8–14 cps) pattern as well as low-amplitude beta (15–35 cps) waves (Figure 2). There may be eye movements, which decrease as the subject begins to fall asleep. Muscle tone is high.

AWAKE

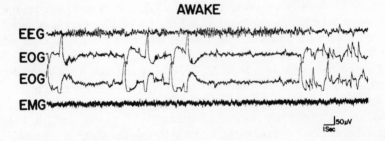

FIGURE 2. Polygraphic recording in an awake young adult. EEG = electroencephalogram; EOG = electrooculogram; EMG = electromyogram.

NonREM Sleep

Stage 1

Alpha activity decreases to less than 50% of each epoch, and the tracing contains a low-voltage mixed-frequency signal with prominent 2- to 7-cps activity; the latter tends to dominate as the subject approaches Stage 2 (Figure 3). There may be slow, "rolling" eye movements. The EMG is somewhat lower in amplitude, indicating that muscle tone is more relaxed than in waking, but there is still substantial muscle tone.

Stage 2

The theta background continues, and on it are superimposed two types of intermittent events: spindles and K complexes (Figure 4). Spindles are rhythmic bursts of 12- to 14-cps waves lasting 0.5 sec or longer. K complexes are high-amplitude waves with a negative and then positive phase, also with a duration of at least 0.5 sec. Sometimes a brief burst of 12- to 14-cps activity may follow the K complex.

STAGE I

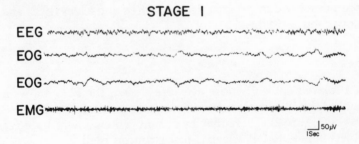

FIGURE 3. Stage 1 sleep.

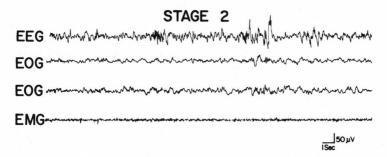

FIGURE 4. Stage 2 sleep.

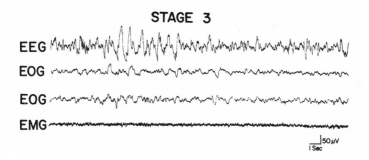

FIGURE 5. Stage 3 sleep.

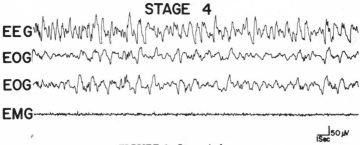

FIGURE 6. Stage 4 sleep.

Stages 3 and 4

These stages are also known as *delta* or *slow-wave* sleep, because they are characterized by high-amplitude (at least 75 μV), slow (0.5- to 2-cps) delta waves. These waves comprise 20–50% of the epoch in Stage 3 (Figure 5), and greater than 50% in Stage 4 (Figure 6). Sleep spindles are sometimes present. Muscle tone is lower in comparison to Stage 1, but a fair amount of tonus is still present.

REM Sleep

This is also referred to as paradoxical sleep or D sleep (Figure 7). The EEG resumes an "activated" pattern similar to Stage 1; REM sleep was often referred to as "Stage 1B" for some years after its discovery). The eyes have rapid conjugate movements. The recording, incidentally, is set up in a manner so that when the eyes move conjugately, the movements of the two eye channels appear as roughly mirror images of each other. The number of eye movements per minute of REM sleep is referred to as the *REM density*. The submental EMG is of greatly decreased amplitude, indicating decreased muscle tone. There are no sleep spindles or K complexes.

An idealized night's sleep in a young adult is pictured in Figure 8. The time from when the lights are turned out until the beginning of sleep is referred to as the *sleep latency*. After sleep onset the sleep stages tend to appear in a rhythmic pattern. In an idealized situation it may be something like this: Stage 1, Stage 2, Stage 3, Stage 4, Stage 3, Stage 2, REM, and then a cyclic repetition of this pattern. This is known as the *REM–nonREM cycle*, which (again in an idealized situation) occurs roughly every 90 min. (There is some reason to believe that this is part of a more fundamental rhythm named by Kleitman, 1963, the "basic rest activity cycle" which occurs around the clock; Broughton, 1973.) Another term which should be noted is the *REM latency*, which is the time from the onset of sleep until the beginning of the first REM sleep period; it is often in the range of 70–90 min in a healthy young adult, but it is decreased in certain illnesses such as narcolepsy (Rechtschaffen, Wolpert, Dement, Mitchell, & Fisher, 1963) and possibly in primary depressive illness (Kupfer, 1976).

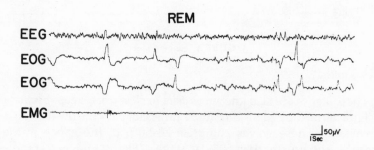

FIGURE 7. REM sleep.

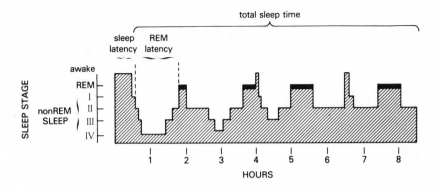

FIGURE 8. An idealized night's sleep in a normal young adult.

INFLUENCES ON THE APPEARANCE OF SLEEP STAGES

As seen in Figure 8, the content of the sleep cycles changes during the period in which one sleeps. There is a tendency for Stages 3 and 4 to occur early in nocturnal sleep, whereas REM sleep tends to be more concentrated after several hours. In a young adult the percentage of nocturnal sleep in each stage is something like this: 50%, Stage 2; 25%, REM sleep; 10%, Stage 3; 10%, Stage 4; 5%, Stage 1. The percentages of the sleep stages very markedly with age (I. Feinberg & Carlson, 1968). During infancy, for instance, there is a great deal of Stage 4 sleep, which then decreases in a hyperbolic curve over adulthood and old age (Figure 9). REM sleep is highest in infancy and childhood, declines but then levels off with maturity, and again declines in old age. Total sleep time follows a similar pattern. The decreased total sleep and increased awakenings during the night in the elderly may be among the reasons leading to their frequent use of hypnotics (see Chapter 9).

Other factors which influence the occurrence of the sleep stages include the duration of wakefulness since the last sleep period and the time of day. The amount of delta sleep, for instance, increases proportionately to the length of the previous period of wakefulness which is inversely related to the sleep latency (Agnew & Webb, 1971). Sleep latency is also influenced by the time at which one goes to sleep; even when the duration of previous wakefulness is constant, one will fall asleep sooner late at night than in the afternoon (Webb & Agnew, 1975). REM sleep is very powerfully affected by the time of day and is much less influenced by prior wakefulness. There is much more REM sleep in the early morning hours than in the afternoon and evening (Weitzman,

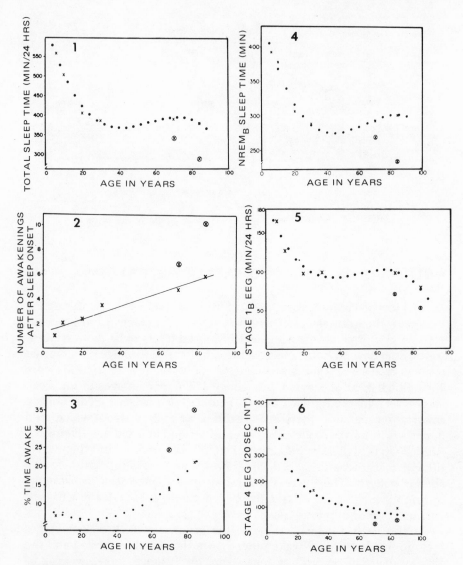

FIGURE 9. Changes in the percentage of the sleep stages with age. (From S. Feinberg & Carlson, 1968, by permission.)

Nogeire, Perlow, Fukushima, Sassin, McGregor, Gallagher, & Hellman, 1974). Naps in the morning, for instance, have much more REM sleep than afernoon naps (Karacan, Williams, Finley, & Hursch, 1970).

These temporal influences on sleep are of course disrupted when one travels by plane to a new time zone, so it is not surprising that travelers should experience difficulty sleeping. It is common practice to take hypnotics when this occurs, but interestingly it is not clear that they are effective in dealing with this problem (see Chapter 4). Other persons may have difficulty sleeping because their rhythm of sleep and wakefulness may differ from that which is most socially acceptable. They may be very comfortable, for instance, going to sleep at 3:00 A.M. and arising at 11:00 A.M., but have great difficulty going to sleep earlier in order to arrive at work at 9:00 A.M. The consequence of this incompatibility of rhythms is known as "phase lag syndrome" and there has been some success in treating it by helping a person progressively to move his hours of sleep later and later until he reaches a more conventional sleep–waking pattern.

There are, then, a number of influences on the onset of sleep and the occurrence of the various sleep stages. Among these are the length of time asleep, the duration of prior wakefulness, an inherent rhythm occurring roughly every 90–100 min, the time of day, and the age of the sleeper. The neurophysiologic bases of these phenomena, which are at best imperfectly understood, will now be reviewed.

PHYSIOLOGIC REGULATION OF SLEEP

Passive versus Active Model

For some time sleep was thought to be an essentially *passive* phenomenon; that is, sensory stimulation was thought to be necessary to stimulate the brain to wakefulness. According to this viewpoint, incoming sensory stimuli not only provide data about the environment but also stimulate an anatomically diffuse network in the brainstem known as the reticular activating system (Moruzzi & Magoun, 1949). This in turn produced wakefulness. It became clear, however, that such a conception was hard pressed to explain a number of findings. These included: (1) the occurrence of two fundamentally different types of sleep (REM and nonREM); (2) observations that electrical stimulation of certain areas of the brain produced sleep; and (3) reports that lesions in the midpontine region resulted in prolonged wakefulness (Jouvet, 1969). In order to deal with these processes, the conception was developed that sleep is an *active* phenomenon, controlled by the interaction of many groups of neurons.

While sleep was thought of as a passive process, it was possible to explain many observations in terms of a "dry" neurophysiology, i.e., purely electrical phenomena. In the passive view, for instance, sleep resulted from such processes as decreased afferent input and neuronal fatigue. The active view, however, encouraged the use of "wet" neurophysiology, the study of the chemical neurotransmitters which carry impulses across the synaptic junction between neurons. This approach, which has been very fruitful, has emphasized the importance of neuron groups containing the biogenic amines and acetylcholine.

The Neurotransmitters

The neuroanatomical areas which have received the most attention as regulators of sleep include the serotonergic cells of the *raphe* nuclei in the midbrain and pons, noradrenergic cells in the *locus coeruleus* of the pons, cholinergic cells in the gigantocellular tegmental field (FTG) of the pons, and dopaminergic cells in the ventral tegmentum of the midbrain (Gillin, Mendelson, Sitaram, & Wyatt, 1978). The precise role of the biogenic animes and acetylcholine is imperfectly understood. A synthesis of available data has suggested that serotonin initiates and maintains nonREM sleep and may play a role in "priming" REM sleep (Jouvet, 1972). The role in nonREM sleep was based on observations that both lesions to the raphe area and the drug parachlorophenylalanine (which blocks serotonin synthesis) greatly decrease total sleep in cats (Jouvet, 1972). Not all investigators confirmed these original observations, however. There is also some evidence that over a period of time sleep tends to return toward normal in such lesioned animals (Morgane & Stern, 1974). The view that serotonin plays a role in priming REM sleep (Jouvet, 1972) is consistent with observations that low doses of parachlorophenylalanine (Wyatt, 1972) or the serotonin receptor blocker methysergide (Mendelson, Reichman, & Othmer, 1975) decrease REM sleep in man, and that low doses of the serotonin precursor 5-hydroxytryptophan (Wyatt, 1972) may increase it. There have also been reports that serotonin-containing neurons may inhibit the appearance of certain phasic events during REM sleep, known as pontine-geniculate-occipital (PGO) spikes (Dement, Mitler, & Henriksen, 1972).

There is some evidence that neurons containing the catecholamines norepinephrine and dopamine may inhibit REM sleep in man. A variety of compounds which might be expected to increase catecholamine activity (e.g., L-dopa, D- and L-amphetamine, methylphenidate, cocaine, peribedil, and clonidine) have been reported to decrease REM sleep (Gillin *et al.*, 1978). Among these, agents that might be expected to stimulate dopamine more than norepinephrine (high doses of L-dopa, D-amphetamine, cocaine) also decrease total sleep, while the norepinephrine agonist clonidine does not. Acute administration of agents that decrease synthesis of catecholamines (alpha-methylparatyrosine; Wyatt,

1972) or block the alpha receptors of norepinephrine (thymoxamine; Oswald, Thacore, Adam, Brezinova, & Burack, 1975) may induce REM sleep. Dopamine receptor blockers such as pimozide (Sagales & Erill, 1975) and chlorpromazine (Sagales, Erill, & Domino, 1969) have much less striking effects.

Lesions of dopaminergic cells in the ventral mesencephalic tegmentum were found to produce akinesia and lack of behavioral arousal which appeared to be in contrast to a waking EEG (Jones, Bobiller, Pin, & Jouvet, 1973). This seemed to suggest a dopaminergic role in the behavioral aspects of arousal. Studies of lesions of the locus coeruleus have been conflicting. Initial results indicated decreases in REM sleep (Jouvet & Delorme, 1965); later work showed no effect on total REM sleep or wakefulness, although fewer PGO spikes occurred (Jones, Harper, & Halaris, 1977). Studies of spontaneous firing of single cells in the cat brainstem suggest that some cells in the locus coeruleus fire rapidly in nonREM sleep and greatly decrease firing during REM sleep. These may function in a complex reciprocal arrangement with cholinergic cells in the FTG field (Hobson, McCarley, & McKenna, 1976). The latter authors observed that in restrained cats the FTG cells fire more rapidly just before REM sleep and during PGO spiking in REM sleep. Subsequent studies by Siegel and McGinty (1977) in freely moving cats have raised the possibility that such firing may not be selective for REM, but also occurs during various kinds of motor activity in unrestrained cats.

Other evidence links the cholinergic system with facilitation of REM sleep. In man and cats, REM sleep may be induced by administering physostigmine, which increases cholinergic activity by blocking its metabolism (Domino, Yamamoto, & Dren, 1968; Sitaram, Wyatt, Dawson, & Gillin, 1976). Conversely, cholinergic blockers such as scopolamine may inhibit REM sleep (Domino et al., 1968), although tolerance to this effect may develop with chronic administration. Lesion studies are not available further to elucidate the role of the cholinergic system because of its more diffuse distribution in the brain. A variety of studies of spontaneous release of acetylcholine, however, also seems to suggest an important role in sleep regulation.

In sum, it seems likely that some aspects of sleep regulation involve the complex interactions of neurons containing biogenic amines and acetylcholine. A number of lines of evidence, including the ability of the nervous system to compensate over a period of time for the immediate changes in sleep induced by acute alterations in these substances, emphasizes the very incomplete and tentative nature of our knowledge. Other aspects of sleep regulation undoubtedly involve other neurotransmitters, perhaps including gamma-aminobutyric acid (GABA) and histamine. There has been much interest in recent years in the role of peptides in the brain (e.g., enkephalins, substance P, somatostatin) as neuroregulators, and their possible role in sleep will have to be explored.

Circulating Humors

There is also evidence that some aspects of sleep may be regulated by circulating substances in the blood. This concept was dramatized in the 19th century by Bouchard, who reported that injections into animals of urine which had been collected during the daytime induced narcosis, while nocturnal urine did not. Such studies were summarized by Hurd (1891), who concluded that "during the period of waking activity the processes of disassimilation give rise to products which by their accumulation cause sleep" (p. 2). Legendre and Pieron reported in 1910 that a material from the cerebrospinal fluid of sleep-deprived dogs could induce sleep when later injected into new animals. Subsequent reports have described such materials from the cerebrospinal fluid of goats (Pappenheimer, Koski, Finch, Karnovsky, & Krueger, 1975), brain extracts from rats (Nagasaki, Iriki, Inone, & Vchizono, 1974), perfusates from the brains of cats (Drucker-Colín & Spanis, 1976), and cerebral venous blood in rabbits (Monnier, Dudler, & Schoenenberger, 1973). One of these substances has been described as a peptide with a molecular weight of 350–500 (Pappenheimer et al., 1975); another has been described as a nonapeptide (Monnier et al., 1977).

One of the difficulties in assessing the physiologic significance of circulating factors is that with few exceptions (Polc, Schneeberger, & Haefely, 1978) the data have not been reported in terms of the traditional sleep staging commonly used in sleep research. Doubts have also been raised by a report showing the independence of sleep patterns in Siamese twins (Lenard & Schulte, 1972) and in a dog with both a natural and a surgically attached head sharing a common circulation (Des Andres, Gutierrez-Rivas, Vava, & Reinoso-Suarez, 1976).

HYPNOTICS AND SLEEP REGULATION

The elaborate neurotransmitter systems described above may be altered by the hypnotics (C.M. Smith, 1977), although it is not clear that this is the mechanism by which they produce their sleep-inducing effects. The barbiturates (see Chapter 3) affect several neurotransmitters; most notably they may inhibit release of acetylcholine (Carmichael & Israel, 1975; Crossland & Slater, 1968) and facilitate some effects of GABA

(Nicoll, 1975a,b). They have also been reported to decrease histamine turnover (Pollard, Bischoff, & Schwartz, 1973, 1974) and to suppress spinal reflex responses to tryptamine (Marley & Vane, 1963). Benzodiazepines (see Chapter 3) may decrease the turnover of norepinephrine, dopamine, and serotonin (Bartholini, Keller, Pieri, & Pletscher, 1973; Taylor & Laverty, 1973; Wise, Berger, & Stein, 1972), and may facilitate the actions of GABA (Costa, Guidotti, & Mao, 1975; Haefely, Kulcsar, Mohler, Pieri, & Schaffner, 1975). There is some interest in the possibility that they act via effects on cyclic AMP (Schultz, 1974a,b), which may alter neuronal functioning. Benzodiazepines may also increase concentrations of acetylcholine, possibly by blocking its release (Consolo, Garattini, & Ladinsky, 1975). There are of course many other mechanisms by which hypnotics may act besides altering the action of neurotransmitters. These include alteration in physical properties of neuron membranes (Seeman, 1975), decreasing cellular energy metabolism (Quastel, 1975), increasing intracellular calcium (Meech, 1972), and other effects.

SLEEP DEPRIVATION

In spite of our growing understanding of sleep regulation and the mechanisms of action of hypnotics, the function of sleep remains a mystery. A classical method of studying the function of a system is to observe the results of depriving an organism of it. This technique—sleep deprivation—has been tried extensively.

There are three basic forms of sleep deprivation. One can deprive a person of all of his sleep (total sleep deprivation), a single stage (selective sleep deprivation), or merely reduce the number of hours of sleep (partial sleep deprivation). Total sleep deprivation for up to 150–200 hr may produce transient psychotic episodes in some persons, but apparently it does not produce lasting harm. This was dramatically brought to public attention in 1959 when Peter Tripp, a New York disc jockey, stayed awake for 200 hr as part of a March of Dimes crusade (Dement, 1973). Tripp, who made a daily broadcast from a booth in Times Square, was observed by researchers including Dr. Jolyan West and Dr. William Dement. Toward the end of his vigil he developed periods of slurred and inappropriate speech, and at night had delusions that enemies were trying surreptitiously to administer sleeping potions to him. Although florid psychotic states develop relatively infrequently (in one study by Tyler in 1955 it occurred in 7 out of 350 subjects deprived of sleep for 112 hr), changes in mood and performance appear regularly in prolonged sleep deprivation.

These may include misinterpretation of stimuli, irritability, and delusions of persecution (Johnson, 1969). Changes in psychological testing have been attributed to decreases in attentiveness (Williams, Lubin, & Goodnow, 1959). During recovery sleep, the proportions of Stage 4 and REM sleep may be increased above baseline values (A. Kales, Tan, Keller, Naitoh, Preston, & Malstrom, 1970).

Sleep deprivation for one night, in contrast to the prolonged deprivation described above, commonly results in complaints of fatigue, irritability, and poor concentration. These are surprisingly difficult to demonstrate consistently with objective testing. There have been reports of increased "sleepiness," "friendliness," and "aggression" (Roth, Kramer, Leston, & Lutz, 1974) as well as "fatigue" and "confusion" (Hartmann, Orzack, & Branconnier, 1974); performance deficits have been attributed to difficulty in encoding new data into short-term memory (Polzella, 1975). In general, decreases in performance after sleep deprivation up to 60 hr are task dependent. As might be expected, more errors are made on complex tasks than on simple ones. The more interesting the task, the better the performance. In fact, the degree of interest may possibly outweigh the effects of the relative complexity of the task (Allnutt & O'Conner, 1971; Wilkinson, 1964).

A subject may be selectively deprived of a sleep stage by awakening him whenever the polygraph indicates that he is entering that stage. This has been done experimentally with both REM sleep (e.g., Clemes & Dement, 1967) and Stage 4 (Agnew, Webb, & Williams, 1964). When a subject is deprived of REM sleep in this manner for several nights, it begins to appear more and more often, and he must be awakened more and more frequently. This is considered to be a manifestation of an increase in a hypothetical *REM pressure.* Upon cessation of REM or Stage 4 deprivation, the recovery sleep may be characterized by a large amount of that stage; this is referred to as a *rebound* phenomenon. A number of drugs including most hypnotics reduce REM sleep, and a REM rebound may be seen during the first few nights after drug administration is terminated. During this period patients often complain of sleep disturbance, which has been attributed by some authors to the increased REM sleep (see Chapter 8). Ethanol also suppresses REM sleep and creates a REM rebound on withdrawal. When chronic alcoholics develop delirium tremens, a psychotic state which may appear during withdrawal, there may be a greatly exaggerated rebound in which REM comprises over 90% of sleep (Chapter 10). REM sleep may also be decreased by getting a subject up every day early in the morning (partial sleep deprivation), since most REM sleep tends to appear in the later hours of nocturnal sleep. Animals may be REM sleep deprived without the necessity of an investigator being in constant attendance to arouse them. They are placed on a small pedestal surrounded by water; the muscle relaxation which accompanies REM sleep leads them to fall into the water, which wakes them up (Mendelson, Guthrie, Frederick, & Wyatt, 1974).

REM sleep deprivation studies have been reviewed by G.W. Vogel (1975). Animal studies have described increased cortical excitability (Owen & Bliss, 1970), aggression (Morden, Connor, Mitchell, Dement, & Levine, 1968), and sexual behavior (Dement, 1965), and impaired memory processes (Fishbein & Gutwein, 1977; Pearlman & Becker, 1974; Stern, 1970). Human REM sleep deprivation studies included initial reports of disturbed or even frankly psychotic behavior after 15 or 16 nights (Dement, 1964), but a variety of later studies failed to confirm these observations (Foulkes, Pivik, Aherns, & Swanson, 1968; A. Kales, Hodemaker, Jacobson, & Lichtenstein, 1964; Snyder, 1963). Thus the effects of REM deprivation are poorly understood. There is even some possibility that it might be beneficial in some circumstances, for instance, as a treatment for depression (G.W. Vogel, 1975; G.W. Vogel, Traub, & Ben-Horin, 1968). It is important to recognize this point because it has been claimed that hypnotics which tend to decrease REM sleep are somehow less desirable than others which often suppress some other aspect of sleep (e.g., slow-wave sleep). Insofar as we have no understanding of the function of any sleep stage, it is clearly too early to base decisions about the desirability of various hypnotics according to which sleep stage they affect most. In principle, an ideal hypnotic might leave the architecture of sleep undisturbed, but such a drug is not yet available.

THE NEED FOR SLEEP

Just as there is little understanding of the functions of sleep, or of individual sleep stages, it is poorly understood how much sleep we "need." It is somewhat easier to get information on how long people tend to sleep, on the assumption that each person somehow "knows" his optimal sleep requirement (Hartmann, 1973). One of the most striking observations is how constant the duration of sleep tends to be despite differences in geographic location, time of sleeping, or societal patterns (Hartmann, 1973). A poll of over one million American adults indicates that the most frequently reported sleep duration is 8.0–8.9 hr, although almost as many younger adults report sleeping 7.0–7.9 hr (Kripke, Simons, Garfinkel, & Hammond, 1979). There is, of course, a wide range around these more typical values. At one extreme are the well-documented cases of "natural short sleepers"—persons who prosper with 3 or 4 hr of sleep per night (H.S. Jones & Oswald, 1968; Meddis, Pearson, & Langford, 1973), whose functioning may actually deteriorate when they get more sleep (Stuss, Healey, & Broughton, 1975). Studies of somewhat less extreme short and long sleepers have not agreed on whether such persons vary in personality traits. Webb and Friel (1971) found no personality or scholastic differences between them. In contrast, Hartmann, Baekland, and Zwilling (1972), and Hartmann (1973), found that short sleepers (who reported sleeping less than 6 hr per night) tended to be "nonworriers," confident and conformist, with little overt psychopathology. Long sleepers (who reported sleeping at least 9 hr per night) tended to be "worriers." They were less conformist, often with psychological and social problems, and sometimes were mildly depressed. Another group, "variable sleepers," seemed to need more sleep at times of stress and less than average sleep at more tranquil times. Insomniacs, in the view of these investigators, differed from all three of these groups, not only because of unhappiness with their sleep, but also in terms of their personality traits. They tended to be more anxious, often displaying mild psychiatric or psychosomatic problems, sometimes characterized by concerns about "losing control" or "letting go."

INSOMNIA

In sum, we know little about the functions of sleep or how much sleep is needed, although we have a fair amount of information on how long people report that they sleep. How difficult it is, then, to find the appropriate treatment for persons who come to the physician complaining that they are sleeping poorly or not getting "enough" sleep. It may be well, then, briefly to discuss what we know (and do not know) about insomnia. The interested reader may also wish to consult a recent compilation of studies in this area (Institute of Medicine, 1979, technical appendix).

Insomnia is primarily a complaint, not an illness. It is characterized by a distressing sensation of inadequate quantity or quality of sleep. Specific complaints (the relative frequencies of which are discussed in Chapter 2) include difficulty going to sleep, multiple awakenings during the night, or early-morning arousals from which it is difficult to return to sleep. In some (the actual percentage is unknown) there is also daytime sleepiness or fatigue. Some patients also complain of "light" sleep, i.e., awakening very easily in response to noises, but they may be a somewhat different group than those who complain of generally poor sleep.*

These various sensations define insomnia at this time because, as we shall see later, objective measures of sleep disturbance in insomniacs have been less helpful than one might anticipate. The quality of distress is important in that it distinguishes insomniacs from the "natural short sleepers" mentioned earlier, who sleep only briefly each night yet feel fine. The quality of daytime fatigue is poorly understood; it has not been clearly demonstrated, for instance, that such uncomfortable individuals actually have objective deficits in daytime performance. From the available data, however, three kinds of findings are beginning to emerge: (1) insomnia is not a simple matter of getting "too little" sleep; (2) the degree of difficulty getting to sleep and the degree of shortened sleep described by insomniacs is usually greater than that which is recorded on the sleep EEG; and (3) insomnia is comprised of a variety of definable conditions which result in a common sensation of having slept poorly. These three points will be considered in turn.

Insomnia and Length of Sleep. Surprisingly, people who complain of insomnia do not get substantially less sleep than those who feel their sleep is adequate. When the total sleep times of 122 insomniacs were compared to normal values in one study, for instance, the insomniacs as a group slept slightly less, but the overlap was substantial (Carskadon, Dement, Mitler, Guilleminault, Zarcone, & Spiegel, 1976). It was found that less than one patient in five who complained of a long sleep latency or short total sleep time had confirmation of this problem by a sleep EEG. In another study of 18 insomniacs and matched controls, the mean difference in sleep time between the two groups was only 43 min, with considerable overlap between them (Frankel, Coursey, Buchbinder, & Snyder, 1976). Thus, although the examination of total sleep time by the EEG may distinguish insomniacs as a group, it has been of little use in diagnosing individual patients. Therefore, until our understanding of insomnia improves, we must rely heavily on the subjective *complaint* of poor sleep rather than objective measures. One hopeful solution to this difficult problem, incidentally, is the possibility that insomniacs can be successfully differentiated from noncomplaining subjects by multivariate analy-

*Rechtschaffen (1969) found that subjects whose overall responses to a questionnaire (Monroe, 1967) categorized them as "good" or "poor" sleepers did not significantly differ in their answers to questions about "light" or "deep" sleep in response to sounds. Conversely, Zimmerman (1967) reported that subjects chosen on the basis of being light or deep sleepers did in fact differ in the ease with which they were aroused by sounds in the laboratory, but had virtually the same responses on the questionnaire for good and poor sleepers.

sis, which characterizes insomniacs by changes in a complex group of sleep variables, rather than by a single trait (Gillin, Duncan, Pettigrew, Frankel, & Snyder, 1979).

The Sensation of Disturbed Sleep. It is apparent that the degree of disturbance described by insomniacs or poor sleepers seems greater than the relatively minor disturbance of sleep recorded by the EEG. This is reflected in several studies in which their estimates of a night's sleep were compared with recorded sleep. Monroe (1967), for instance, found that poor sleepers* estimated that it took them 59 min to fall asleep, while the EEG sleep latency was 15 min. In contrast, the good sleepers estimated that it usually took them 7 min to fall asleep, which is precisely what was reported by the EEG. On the other hand, the poor sleepers did not seem to exaggerate all their difficulties—they actually underestimated the number of times they awakened during the night. In a study of insomniacs (from which patients with sleep apnea and nocturnal myoclonus had been excluded), the patients reported a total sleep time of 332.8 min, although the EEG indicated 375.0 min (Carskadon *et al.*, 1976). The insomniacs estimated that their sleep latency was 61.7 min, although the mean EEG value was 26.2 min. As in the Monroe study of poor sleepers, the insomniacs also *underestimated* their number of arousals, suggesting that perhaps they do not exaggerate all their disturbances. Similar results were reported by Frankel *et al.* (1976), although they did not observe the underestimation of arousals (Figure 10). Interestingly, although these studies indicated differences in the insomniacs' subjective estimate and recorded value for sleep latency and total sleep, the report and the objective measure did correlate significantly.

It is not clear what leads insomniacs to exaggerate their degree of difficulty in falling asleep or in achieving a long duration of sleep. One possibility is that the act of lying in bed unable to sleep is very distressing, lending itself to be the natural tendency to exaggerate the extent of uncomfortable experiences (Frankel *et al.*, 1976). Another possibility is

---

*Monroe (1967) found subjects by administering questionnaires about sleep habits and subjective experience of sleeping to 200 persons in a university community, and selecting from among them 16 "good" sleepers and 16 "poor sleepers." It is important to note, then, that they "cannot be considered an extremely sleep-disturbed group; none of the poor sleepers perceived themselves 'as being insomniacs' or as having any specific type of sleep disturbance" (p. 257). The point, then, is that these were persons who clearly were unhappy with their sleep but may have had a relatively mild disturbance. As the type of subject may very much influence the results of treatment studies (see Chapter 4), it is important to bear in mind when subjects are obtained by questionnaire and when they come from those who seek medical help. Many studies of autonomic activity and effects of relaxation-inducing treatments (Chapter 11), for instance, employed subjects obtained by administering questionnaires to psychology students.

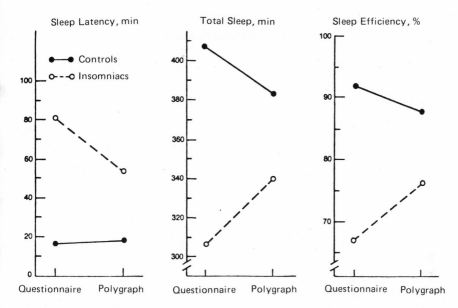

FIGURE 10. Comparison of questionnaire and EEG sleep variables of insomniacs and control subjects. (From Frankel *et al.*, 1976, by permission).

that persons who sleep poorly differ in their degree of arousal during EEG-defined sleep. Rechtschaffen (1969), for instance, reported that when an investigator entered the room of persons who were asleep by EEG criteria (10 min after the first spindle), poor sleepers often (6 out of 22 awakenings) said that they had actually been awake, while this happened only once among the good sleepers. The poor sleepers frequently described more thought-like processes when awakened by investigators than did the good sleepers. Thus one might speculate that people who sleep poorly are accurately reflecting some difference in the degree of self-awareness during sleep.

Many Causes for One Sensation. It is becoming clear that a sizable percentage of persons who complain of poor sleep have diagnosable conditions of which they may be unaware. Among these are the sleep apnea syndromes, nocturnal myoclonus, depressive illness, and the phase lag syndrome which was mentioned earlier (see Table I). What these conditions all have in common is that they somehow produce the sensation of having slept poorly. It is important to bear this in mind, because it means that one cannot meaningfully evaluate treatments for "insomnia" or study differences between "insomniacs" and noncomplaining subjects without considering the possible presence of several different associated conditions.

TABLE I
Disorders Associated with Insomnia[a]

DISORDERS OF INITIATING AND MAINTAINING SLEEP (DIMS)

1. Psychophysiological. These include transient situational disturbances (e.g., sleeping in a strange place, bereavement, anxiety associated with changing jobs) as well as more persistent sleep disturbances which seemed to start in this manner.

2. Psychiatric Disturbances. These include insomnia associated with character disorders, neuroses, schizophrenia and affective disorders. Among patients with clear psychiatric illness, the incidence of sleep disturbance is very high, occurring for instance in 72% of outpatients in one study (Weiss, Kasinoff, & Bailey, 1962). In depressive illness, sleep time is markedly decreased and early-morning awakenings are increased compared to control subjects (Gillin *et al.*, 1979). Decreased sleep also often accompanies acute exacerbations of schizophrenia (Snyder, 1969). Polygraphic studies of sleep in these conditions have recently been reviewed (Mendelson, Gillin, & Wyatt, 1977).

Studies of groups of insomniacs who had not been selected on the basis of psychiatric illness have rather consistently noted a high incidence of abnormal scores on the Minnesota Multiphasic Personality Inventory (MMPI), especially the depression, hysteria, and hypochondriasis scales (Carskadon *et al.*, 1976; Coursey, Buchsbaum, & Frankel, 1975; Monroe, 1967; Roth & Krammer, 1975).[b] Such findings have led a number of authors to emphasize the role of depressed mood or anxious, worrying personality traits in insomnia (Coursey *et al.*, 1975; Hartmann, 1973). It is not clear, of course, whether such traits are a cause or result of insomnia, or whether both are manifestations of some other process.

3. Use of Drugs and Alcohol. Included here is the persistent sleep disturbance which sometimes occurs in patients who develop tolerance to hypnotics and seek relief in progressively larger doses (Chapter 8). There is also frequently a transient withdrawal insomnia which occurs when treatment with traditional doses of many hypnotics is discontinued (Chapter 8). Alcoholics, even when "dry," have disturbed sleep characterized by increased arousals and changes between sleep stages, and decreased slow-wave sleep (Chapter 10). Some authors have commented that these persistent sleep changes are similar to the characteristics of sleep in the elderly (J.W. Smith, Johnson, & Burdick, 1971). Sleep disturbance may also appear in patients who are chronically taking stimulants.

4. Sleep-Induced Ventilatory Impairment. Most important here are the sleep apnea syndromes (Guilleminault & Dement, 1978), of which there are three types: central, mixed, and obstructive. In central sleep apnea, there are multiple (70–300) apneic episodes lasting 10 sec to 3 min, due to a failure of the nervous system to stimulate diaphragmatic movement. These episodes are often terminated by brief awakenings, the cumulative effect of which may be disturbed sleep. In "mixed" sleep apnea, there are in addition transient periods of upper airway obstruction due to relaxation of the pharyngeal musculature. During these episodes the diaphragm contracts vigorously in an effort to move air, resulting in loud snoring. This latter situation occurs alone in "obstructive" sleep apnea, which is often associated with excessive daytime sleepiness. During apneic episodes, oxygen saturation plummets and asystoles may occur. In the long term, obstructive sleep apnea may be associated with the development of pulmonary and sometimes systemic hypertension. It is also worrisome in that administration of hypnotics may further compromise the respiration of sleep apnea patients, with potentially hazardous consequences.

The frequency of central sleep apnea is not known. Although one clinic found none among 72 patients complaining of insomnia (Bixler, Saldatos, Kales, & Russek, 1976), others have reported frequencies of 12% (Dement, Guilleminault, & Zarcone, 1975b), 6% (Hauri, 1976) and 5% (Billiard, Besset, & Passousant, 1976). Central sleep apnea is thought to be more common in men than women, most frequently over 40. There is some tentative evidence from Stanford University that the incidence may be much higher in the elderly both among noncomplaining individuals and those with sleep disturbance (Institute of Medicine, 1979).

There is no clear treatment for central sleep apnea, although some promising work with chlorimipramine has been done. Obstructive sleep apneas may be successfully treated with a chronic tracheostomy which is opened at night.

5. *Nocturnal Myoclonus and the "Restless Legs Syndrome."* The former condition is characterized by brief (0.5–4.0 sec) clonic movements of one or both legs, occurring as often as every 20–40 sec. These may be accompanied on the EEG by a K complex, a brief burst of alpha activity, or a brief awakening. The patient is often completely unaware of these episodes, and history is best elicited from a bed partner. This is not an epileptic phenomenon.

In one clinic series, nocturnal myoclonus appeared in 17% of insomniac patients (Dement, Guilleminault, & Zarcone, 1975a). One group found nocturnal myoclonic movements no more frequent in insomniacs than controls and has suggested that this is not an important causative factor in insomnia (Bixler, Soldatos, Scarone, Martin, Kales, & Charney, 1978). On the other hand, it has been reported so frequently by many clinics that a final outcome will have to await further studies. There is some possibility, of course, that although both noncomplaining subjects and insomniacs have myoclonic movements in sleep, some quality of the latter group makes them more subject to arousal in response to these movements. There is also some suggestion that nocturnal myoclonus occurs as frequently in those who complain of excessive daytime sleepiness as those who complain primarily of insomnia (Zorich, Roth, Salio, Kramer, & Lutz, 1978). Because it has been found in a variety of disorders, some have speculated that chronic sleep disturbance leads to nocturnal myoclonus, as well as vice versa.

There is no clearly effective treatment for nocturnal myoclonus. Some groups (e.g., Billiard, Besset, & Passouant, 1978) use 5-hydroxytryptophan, while others (Guilleminault, Spiegel, & Dement, 1977) have seen no benefit; the latter group has reported slight improvement with diazepam (Guilleminault *et al.*, 1977).

The "restless legs" syndrome, which may occur either in combination with nocturnal myoclonus or alone, has been reported by a number of authors since the description by Willis in the 17th century. It consists of an uncomfortable sensation of the legs, which starts when the limbs are at rest and is relieved only by constant movement (Frankel, Patten, & Gillin, 1974). This is not necessarily related to anxiety and may occur while the subject is relaxed; in fact, it often seems to become worse when going to sleep. Although sometimes associated with neurologic findings, it often occurs in a patient with a completely normal neurological exam. A case report suggested that 5-hydroxytryptophan may be of benefit (Guilleminault *et al.*, 1977).

6. *Associated with Other Medical, Toxic, and Environmental Conditions.* Sleep disturbance is of course a common problem accompanying medical illnesses. It may be related to pain, or to more specific processes which disturb sleep (nocturnal postural dyspnea in cardiac patients or awakenings to urinate in patients with diabetes mellitus). When alcoholics stop drinking there may occur a withdrawal syndrome, such as delirium tremens, during which sleep is

Continued

TABLE I (Continued)

very disturbed (Chapter 10). Parasomnias (e.g., bruxism, enuresis, sleepwalking) are also classified here when they are associated with sleep disturbance.

7. Childhood Onset. Relatively little is known about insomnia in childhood. A Japanese study which screened the health of 3-year-olds noted its frequency and showed a significant relationship between a parental history of childhood sleep difficulties and its occurrence in their children (Abe & Shimakawa, 1966). More attention is now being focused on insomnia in adolescents, which was found to be a chronic problem in 12.6% in one study (Price, Coates, Thoreson, & Grinstead, 1978).

8. Other DIMS Conditions. These include sleep disturbance with atypical features on polygraphic recordings and repeated awakenings during REM sleep. This later phenomenon was described by Greenberg (1967) among patients who reported multiple awakenings (every hour or so) throughout the night, and who usually had a history of nightmares before developing insomnia.

9. No DIMS Abnormality. Included here are the "natural short sleepers" mentioned previously, as well as the many persons who complain of disturbed sleep but who have no objective findings (as we understand them at this time) on the sleep EEG (see Chapters 1 and 4).

DYSSOMNIAS ASSOCIATED WITH DISRUPTIONS OF 24-HOUR SLEEP–WAKE CYCLE

The importance of sleep as a biological rhythm has been discussed in Chapter 1. An acute "phase shift" in sleep may result from rapid travel across time zones, or by a changing-shift work schedule. Some patients may have a fixed-phase shift in which they tend to go to bed in the middle of the night and get up in the late morning, but have great difficulty conforming to more traditional hours. This may be accompanied by a 24-hr temperature curve which also suggests a lag in the normal circadian rhythm (normally the lowest temperature is at roughly 6:00 A.M. and the highest is in the afternoon; in these patients the peak may be shifted to a later time). Primarily evidence suggests that such patients may be treated by having them go to sleep an hour later each night until more conventional hours are achieved.

Other patients in this category are those whose "natural" sleep–wake rhythm is longer or shorter than 24 hr, and those with irregular sleep–wake patterns. In one case series, circadian rhythm disturbances accounted for 10% of patients complaining of insomnia (Dement *et al.*, 1975b).

---

[a]This classification is adapted from the Nosology Committee of the Association of Sleep Disorder Centers, also subsequently published in modified form (Institute of Medicine, 1979). It has not yet been fully tested in extensive case series, and should be considered tentative and subject to change with experience. Some relevant references and comments by this author are provided. This is intended as a brief guide; the interested reader is encouraged to consult the complete ASDC nosology.

[b]It should be noted that the MMPI contains a number of questions about sleep, which may have influenced this finding. Another possibility rasied by Monroe (1967) is that the pathological scores of poor sleepers represent a "differential response bias," in which they are more likely to subscribe to symptomatic complaints on testing.

SUMMARY AND CONCLUSIONS

There are thought to be three fundamental states of consciousness—waking, REM sleep, and nonREM sleep. The latter is subdivided into four stages. Their occurrence is influenced by a variety of factors including the age of the subject, time of day, time since the last sleeping period, duration of sleep, and a roughly 90- to 100-min sleep cycle which may be part of a more basic rest-activity cycle. The regulation of sleep is an active process which seems to involve the interaction of groups of neurons using a variety of neurotransmitters, including the biogenic amines and acetylcholine. It is less clear what function is served by having such elaborate mechanisms for sleep, and how much sleep one "needs." Insomnia, which involves the sensation of inadequate quantity or quality of sleep, is clearly not just a matter of getting less than average amount of sleep and is often the result of various definable related disorders. It is, then, a complex problem, not given to simple therapeutic solutions.

CHAPTER 2

The Prevalence of Sleep Disturbance and Hypnotic Use

Now if insomnia is going to be one of your naturals, it begins to appear in the late thirties. Those seven previous hours of sleep suddenly break in two. There is, if one is lucky, the "first sweet sleep of night" and the last deep sleep of morning, but between the two appears a sinister, ever widening interval.
—F. Scott Fitzgerald, *Sleeping and Waking*

SURVEYS OF REPORTED SLEEP DISTURBANCE

A variety of studies suggest that a high proportion of Americans are dissatisfied with their sleep (Table II). Balter and Bauer (1975), for instance, found that 11% of men and 17% of women felt that they had "a lot of trouble" getting to sleep or staying asleep, while an additional 19% reported milder degrees of the same complaints. A survey sponsored by the American Cancer Society, in which over one million men and women were interviewed in 1959 and 1960, found that 13.0% of men and 26.4% of women complained of "insomnia" (Hammond, 1964). Studies of populations in more restricted areas such as San Francisco (Welstein, Dement, & Mitler, 1978), Los Angeles (A. Kales, Bixler, Leo, Healy, & Slye, 1974), Houston (Thornby, Karacan, Searle, Salis, Ware, & Williams, 1977), Alachua County, Florida (Karacan, Thornby, Anch, Holzer, Warheit, Schwab, & Williams, 1976), and St. Louis (Brownman, Gordon,

TABLE II. Surveys of Reported Sleep

Author	Location	Number of subjects	Prevalence of sleep complaint
Balter & Bauer, 1975 (National Survey on Drug Acquisition and Use, 1970–1971)	National	2552 (1502 women & 1050 men) aged 18–74 in educational or social organizations	11% M. and 17% F. had "trouble getting to sleep" in the past 12 months and indicated that this was "a lot of trouble"; an additional 19% had a sleep problem that was "not much trouble."
F.C. Hammond, 1964, and Kripke et al., 1979	National	1,064,004 (602,564 women & 461,440 men) from 30 to over 85	13.0% men and 26.4% of women had "insomnia."
Welstein et al., 1978, and Institute of Medicine, 1979	San Francisco area	6352	38% answered "yes" to questions about difficulty going to sleep, awakening during the night or early in the morning; only 4% felt that they had "insomnia."
Kales, Bixler, Leo, Healy, & Slye, 1974	Los Angeles	1000 households	32.2% had a "complaint" of insomnia (14.4% had trouble falling asleep, 22.8% had trouble waking up during the night, and 13.7% had early-morning awakening in these overlapping groups); male/female ratio of complaint of insomnia was similar to population sample.
Karacan et al., 1976	Alachua County, Fla.	1645 adults over 18	35.4% reported a sleep disturbance (22.0% sometimes and 13.4% often or all the time); of those with a sleep disturbance, the most common (55%) complaint was taking too long to go to sleep; no difference between blacks and whites.

Disturbance and Hypnotic Use

Relationship of reported sleep disturbance to age	Use of hypnotics	Comment
For women, prevalence of sleep disturbance increased with age. For men, there was a higher prevalence for those over 60 and under 30. Under age 30, men and women had a roughly equal proportion of major sleep problems, but at older ages, women exceeded men.	In the past year, 3% of men and 4% of women had used a prescription hypnotic and 6% of men and women used a nonprescription hypnotic; 23% of the prescription hypnotic users (about 1% of the population) used them heavily (daily use for at least 2 months); only 2% of nonprescription users took them heavily.	
Increase with age in both sexes.	1.4% of men and 2.5% of women used hypnotics "often" while 10.4% and 18.6%, respectively, took them "seldom" (figures on hypnotic use exclude subjects with history of heart disease, high blood pressure, diabetes, or stroke).	Complex relationship between insomnia and sleeping pill use, e.g., some persons took hypnotics "often," but "seldom" had insomnia.
		Of those persons with complaints about their sleep, only 19.5% sought help from a doctor.
Increase in complaints of sleep disturbance with age; younger males were less likely to complain and older females were more likely to.	20.7% of the 32.2% who complained of sleep disturbance (6% of the sample) used hypnotics at least several times a month; no significant differences in hypnotic use between men and women.	Waking up during night occurred significantly more often by itself than the other complaints alone or in combination.
Increased with age.	7.1% "sometimes" and 3.4% "often" or "all the time"; was higher in women than men, increased with age, and was higher in the divorced, widowed, or separated.	

Continued

TABLE II

Author	Location	Number of subjects	Prevalence of sleep complaint
Thornby et al., 1977	Houston	3 samples: (1) 2347 adults over 18 yrs. (2) 110 couples (3) 293 Mexican-Americans	33% of all three samples had difficulty getting to sleep at least "sometimes"; 48% of major sample reported awakening during night at least sometimes; 22% of all three samples reported early-morning awakenings at least "sometimes"; sleeping difficulty inversely related to education; housewives had more trouble than other occupations; no differences between blacks and whites; sleeping difficulties more common in women than men.
Brownman et al., 1977	St. Louis	365 blue-collar workers (63.5% male), 19–65 yr old	26.7% reported often having difficulty falling asleep or staying asleep; no sex differences.
McGhie & Russell, 1962	Dundee and Glascow, Scotland	2446, aged 15 to over 75 in educational or social organizations	Difficulty going to sleep varied from about 4% in men age 15 to about 10% in men age 75 and over; in women it increased markedly from about 2% at 15 to 30% at 65; frequent awakenings rises in men from 4% at 15 to 35% at 65; lower social classes have more trouble with going to sleep and light sleep, but less morning tiredness.[a]

[a] Percentage estimated from graphs.

Tepas, & Walsh, 1977) reported that approximately one-third to one-half of individuals are unhappy about the quality of their sleep. In most, but not all (A. Kales, Bixler, Leo, Healy, & Slye, 1974) cases, reports of poor sleep have been more frequent among women than men, and in all studies there has been an increased prevalence with advancing age (e.g., Figure 11). There is some reason to think that disturbed sleep is reported more often with descending socioeconomic status (Thornby et al., 1977; McGhie & Russell, 1962; Thornby et al., 1977; Weiss et al., 1962). It may be

(Continued)

Relationship of reported sleep disturbance to age	Use of hypnotics	Comment
Increased with age.	9.7% at least "sometimes"; use of hypnotics inversely related to education and income levels; higher in housewives, executives, tense persons.	
With increasing age there is reduction in total sleep, increased sleep latency, tendency for sleep to be "light," and increased awakenings; morning tiredness does not increase with age; daytime tiredness increased only after age 75.	Prescription hypnotics taken habitually, in men: 5% at age 15, 25% at age 75; in women: 5% at age 15, 45% at age 75; not affected by social class.[a]	

more common among the divorced, widowed, and separated (Clift, 1975b; Karacan *et al.*, 1976; Thornby *et al.*, 1977) and in pregnant (Karacan, Heine, Agnew, Williams, Webb, & Ross, 1968; Schweiger, 1972) and postmenopausal (C.B. Ballinger, 1976) women. Psychiatric patients seem to be particularly vulnerable, with reports of poor sleep in 63–72% of outpatients (Sweetwood, Kripke, Grant, Yager, & Gerst, 1976; Weiss *et al.*, 1962) and perhaps 80% of inpatients (Detre, 1966).

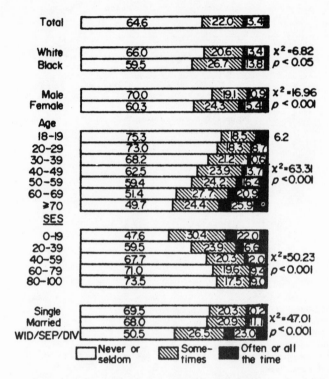

FIGURE 11. Responses to the question "How often do you have trouble sleeping?" (From a study in Alachua County, Florida, by Karacan *et al.*, 1976, by permission.)

TYPES OF SLEEP COMPLAINTS

As mentioned in Chapter 1, complaints about sleep have traditionally been divided into three groups described by Kleitman (1963): trouble going to sleep, awakening during the night, or early-morning awakening. The relative prevalence of these problems is not clear. A. Kales, Bixler, Leo, Healy, & Slye (1974) and Thornby *et al.* (1977), found that among those who reported sleep disturbances, awakening during the night was the most common complaint. Karacan *et al.* (1976), on the other hand, found that 55% of those with complaints about their sleep were concerned with difficulty falling asleep, while only 15% complained of awakenings during the night. Guilleminault *et al.* (1977) found that the most common single complaint among 549 insomniacs was trouble going to sleep, although many were troubled also by nocturnal awakenings. Welstein *et al.* (1978), on the other hand, found that among women the complaints were rather equally divided among these three sleep symptoms and daytime tiredness (a symptom which has probably not received enough attention); among men, problems of early-morning awakening were slightly more common.

From these legions of unhappy persons come frequent requests to physicians for pharmacologic relief (most often, as we shall see later, in the context of coming to the office for another reason). For this and other reasons, physicians issued perhaps 26 million prescriptions for hypnotics in 1977 (Institute of Medicine, 1979), and in addition gave substantial amounts to hospitalized or institutionalized patients. People also treat themselves, by purchasing 30 million packages of nonprescription ("over-the-counter" or OTC) sleep aids annually (Product Marketing, 1978), as discussed in Chapter 10. The consequences of this widespread consumption of hypnotics, which are the subject of this book, are best understood after reviewing the extent of hypnotic use. This can be approached several different ways; including: (1) population surveys; (2) analyses of how patients obtain hypnotic prescriptions from physicians; and (3) analyses of the number of prescriptions written annually. Each of these will be examined in turn.

SURVEYS OF HYPNOTIC USE

The extent of hypnotic use and its relation to the complaint of insomnia was analyzed by Kripke et al. (1979), using data from a study by the American Cancer Society, mentioned earlier (Hammond, 1964). (Other data from this study, such as the relation of cigarette smoking to cancer and heart disease, are well known.) In this particular analysis, they eliminated subjects with histories of heart disease, high blood pressure, diabetes, and stroke, leaving about 750,000 persons. It was found that 1.4% of men and 2.5% of women reported using hypnotics "often," and an additional 10.4% and 18.6% reported using them "seldom." There was some association between the complaint of insomnia and the use of sleeping pills (28% of subjects who had insomnia "often" took hypnotics "often"). On the other hand, 33% of the women and 50% of the men who took hypnotics often reported little or no trouble with insomnia. [One explanation for this might be that in the popular mind "insomnia" is a term reserved for a particularly severe sleep disturbance; as can be seen in several studies, e.g., Welstein et al. (1978), many people complain of various difficulties sleeping, but do not characterize themselves as insomniacs.] Subjects were also asked how long they usually slept. Hypnotic use was greater among those who reported sleeping less than 7 hr, but the report of short sleep related more closely to the complaint of insomnia than to the use of hypnotics. Those complaining of insomnia reported sleeping about an hour less than noncomplaining subjects, but many of their values were well within the normal range of sleep times. Those who had insomnia often and took hypnotics often also reported somewhat shorter sleep durations than those with no sleep complaints or pill use, but once again there was a great deal of overlap. (One possibility, of course, is that they sleep this long *because* they are taking sleeping pills.) This seems to point once again to the complexity of the problems with which we are dealing: insomniacs, whether or not they are taking hypnotics, do not necessarily report sleeping less than others. Another aspect of this particular study was the association of hypnotic use and increased mortality. Those who reported using hypnotics "often" were 1.5 times more likely to die during the next 6 years, even though they had no prior history of heart disease, hypertension, diabetes, or stroke. Although these data are associational and do not necessarily imply causality, they raise the possibility that the widespread hypnotic use described in this section may be related to public health problems more far reaching than those usually considered.

Parry, Balter, Mellinger, Cisin, & Manheimer (1973) and Balter and Bauer (1975), whose report on complaints of sleep disturbance in 2552 adults has already been mentioned, found that 3% of men and 4% of women surveyed in 1970–1971 had taken prescription hypnotics in the past year and that an additional 6% had taken OTC hypnotics. This nearly equal sex ratio is in contrast to the use of prescription psychotherapeutic drugs as a whole, which are consumed by twice as many women as men (29% versus 13%). In use of all OTC drugs and OTC hypnotics, the percentages of men and women were about equal. For both sexes, the use of prescription hypnotics increased with age. The tendency was for approximately equal proportions (1% each) to consume prescription hypnotics at high (daily for 6 months or more), medium, and low rates.

Karacan et al. (1976), in the study of Alachua County, found that 7.1% of subjects used hypnotics "sometimes" and an additional 3.4% took them "often" or "all the time." Use of hypnotics was more common in women than men (13.6% versus 6.7%), and increased markedly with age. (Before age 29 men and women used them about equally, and after 29 women predominated.) Single persons used hypnotics the least (5.8% sometimes or more often) while widowed, divorced, or separated individuals had the most (15.6%).

A survey sponsored by the National Institute on Drug Abuse (NIDA)

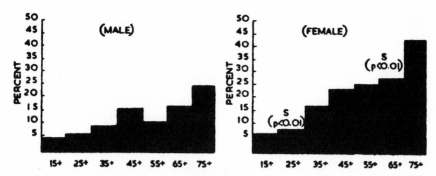

FIGURE 12. Prevalence of persons "in the habit of taking a hypnotic" in a Scottish study. (From McGhie & Russell, 1962, by permission.)

examined the use of hypnotics* in a national sample which included 3322 adults over 18 years old (Abelson, Fishburne, & Cisin, 1977). They found that 8.7% had used such agents for medical purposes in the past year, about half of which was during the last month. As in previous studies (e.g., Figure 12) there was an increased frequency of use with age and a somewhat higher prevalence among women (10%) than men (8%). Like the Alachua County study, which reported no difference in hypnotic use among different socioeconomic groups, the Abelson study indicated similar usage in college graduates and subjects without a high school diploma. There was also no difference between metropolitan and non-metropolitan areas in usage during the past year.

Guilleminault *et al.* (1977) interviewed 549 self-described insomniacs in Los Angeles in 1973, and found that about two-thirds took "pills" (usually prescription hypnotics) at least occasionally, and 40% of the total group took them frequently. About one in five used daytime napping as a way of dealing with their insomnia. (This was particularly common in the elderly.) Many others dealt with their distress by using ethanol (see Chapter 7), while others took over-the-counter hypnotics. There are, then, a number of ways in which persons seek relief from disturbed sleep. It might be well to discuss briefly the option of going to a physician, and how physicians respond to this problem.

PATIENT–PHYSICIAN INTERACTION

In a population study of 6352 subjects in San Francisco, only 19.5% of persons who complained of disturbed sleep consulted a physician (Wel-

---

*These data also include barbiturates often used for daytime sedation (phenobarbital and butabarbital).

stein *et al.*, 1978). Of these, only one in five did so primarily because of the sleep disturbance. Similarly, a nationwide analysis of office practice found that only in 0.3% of visits did the patient come with a primary complaint of sleep disturbance [National Center for Health Statistics (NCHS)] (This relative infrequency of primary complaint of sleep disturbances, which more commonly arise in the context of discussion of a medical or psychiatric illness, may influence how physicians come to view sleep disorders.)

In contrast to the relative infrequency with which patients go to a physician for relief of disturbed sleep, hypnotic prescriptions are written fairly often. Among explanations for this disparity might be: (1) that physicians and patients most commonly discuss sleep problems (and produce prescriptions) in the context of some other illness; and (2) that hypnotics are prescribed for some other purpose than aiding sleep. There is probably some truth in both of these hypotheses. In 1977, a sleep disturbance was considered the primary diagnosis in only 15% of office visits in which a hypnotic was prescribed (National Disease and Therapeutic Index).* By far the most common diagnoses were mental disorders (34%), including most often neurotic depressive reactions (11%) and anxiety reactions (8%). Other disorders included circulatory problems (13%), "special conditions without sickness" (7%), disorders of bones and organs of movement (5%), respiratory (4%), and other disorders (18%). In only 71% of the cases did the physicians state that the desired result of the hypnotic prescription was to improve sleep (NDTI). Other reasons included daytime sedation (5%), pain relief (1%), and other reasons (3%) including symptomatic relief and lowering blood pressure. In 20% of the cases, physicians did not report a reason when prescribing a hypnotic, implying perhaps a general (but vague) feeling that their use was somehow appropriate.

Reflecting the observation that mental disorders were the most common diagnoses when hypnotics were prescribed, the data suggest that psychiatrists prescribe hypnotics disproportionately more frequently than most other specialties. Although they handled only about 3% of the office visits, they wrote 23% of hypnotic prescriptions (NDTI). In contrast, general and family practitioners, who accounted for 33% of office

---

*Data for the National Disease and Therapeutic Index (NDTI), conducted by IMS America, Ltd., is collected from a representative group of 525 physicians who four times a year report on all the prescriptions they write in a 48-hr period. For each prescription they record the drug, demographic information about the patient, diagnosis, whether the therapy is new or ongoing, and other data. All data cited from this source and from the National Prescription Audit (NPA), which estimates the annual number of prescriptions for various drugs, are derived from the Institute of Medicine (1979) report or NIDA Capsules (1978).

visits, and internists (11%), wrote prescriptions roughly proportionate to the number of visits they handled. The family physicians and internists seemed to prescribe barbiturate hypnotics somewhat more often than other hypnotics. In contrast, psychiatrists prescribed nonbarbiturates (largely flurazepam) twice as often as barbiturate hypnotics.

PRESCRIPTIONS FOR OUTPATIENTS

When we examine the total number of prescriptions for hypnotics coming from office visits to physicians, the most obvious trend is that they are declining. In 1971 there were approximately 43 million prescriptions for all hypnotics, compared to approximately 26 million in 1977 (NPA). In addition, roughly 5 million prescriptions for nonhypnotic medications (antidepressants, anxiolytics, antihistamines) were written with the primary intention of aiding sleep (NDTI). (It seems likely that in many more cases where anxiolytics were given with a primary intention other than aiding sleep, doses are frequently given several times a day, including bedtime.) The declining number of hypnotic prescriptions parallels data from the National Institute of Drug Abuse (NIDA)-sponsored population study which indicated that medical use of sedatives in the past year dropped from 11% in 1972 to 8.7% in 1977 (Abelson et al., 1977). There is no evidence to suggest that this decrease is offset by greater use of anxiolytics. The number of prescriptions for anxiolytics has remained relatively constant, at 89 million in 1971 and 90 million in 1977 (NDTI). Similarly, patient usage has remained at about 27% annually, from 1972 to 1977 (Abelson et al., 1977). In order to give a sense of proportion to the number of prescriptions, it should be noted that all 1977 hypnotic prescriptions combined were slightly less than those for antidepressants (30 million), less than half of the number for the anxiolytic diazepam (54 million), and only somewhat greater than those for the analgesic D-propoxyphene (19 million). During this period of 39% decline in all hypnotic prescriptions, there was a disproportionate (77%) decrease in hypnotic barbiturate prescriptions. A variety of nonbarbiturate hypnotics (e.g., chloral hydrate glutethimide, methyprylon, ethchlorvynol, methaqualone) prescriptions also declined by 50–80%. In contrast, there has been a remarkable increase in the prescribing of flurazepam. In 1971 flurazepam comprised 7% of hypnotic prescriptions; this rose annually to 53% in 1977.

Hypnotic prescriptions are usually written for 1 month or longer. During the period from May 1976 to April 1977, the average flurazepam prescription was for 31 capsules; for other nonbarbiturates the range was 32–40, while hypnotic barbiturate prescriptions average 45–91 pills (NPA).

PRESCRIBING HYPNOTICS IN HOSPITAL PRACTICE

Although national data are lacking, and some of the most complete studies are not as current as might be desired, all indications are that a very high percentage—perhaps half—of all hospitalized patients receive hypnotics. In a survey of 4177 patients in three Boston hospitals, Shapiro, Sloan, Lewis, & Jick (1969) reported that 49% received one or more of the four most commonly used hypnotics (chloral hydrate, diphenhydramine, secobarbital, or pentobarbital). Similarly, Morrison and Mayfield (1972), examining medical and surgical patients at the Veterans Administration hospital in Durham, found that 41–54% received hypnotics, and that orders for their use had been written for 66–92%, usually to be given PRN (as needed). On average, they received hypnotics 6.2–9.5 nights per month. The highest percentage of hypnotic orders and administration was in the surgical specialties, followed by general surgery and medicine. In a Glasgow general hospital, 28% of patients received a hypnotic during their stay (Kesson, Gray, & Lawson, 1976). Drug Enforcement Administration reports for the Boston Hospital for Women found that there were 0.40 doses per patient-day on an obstetrical service and 0.30 for gynecologic inpatients during 1974–1975 (Kaul, Harsfield, Osathanondh, & Ostheimer, 1978). (Since diazepam and flurazepam would not be on these reports, the actual number of patients who received drugs for sleep was probably even higher.) Studies of institutionalized geriatric patients show extremely high levels of routine use of hypnotics, varying from 26% (Martilla, Hammel, Alexander, & Zustiak, 1977), to 50% (Mulligan & O'Grady, 1971) to 100% (Derbez & Grauer, 1967). This high incidence of prescribing for the elderly is of particular concern because of their increased susceptibility to side effects, a subject discussed in detail in Chapter 9. The widespread prescribing to inpatients carries another implication. Administration of hypnotics to acutely hospitalized medical patients is one of the most widely accepted uses of hypnotics. Thus medical students and young physicians, whose training occurs largely with such patients, start their medical careers in a setting in which critical thinking is not usually applied to the decision to prescribe hypnotics.

SUMMARY AND CONCLUSIONS

A high percentage of Americans—perhaps one-third—report disturbed sleep and perhaps one-third of these unhappy individuals find it a major problem. Sleep disturbance is generally more common in women, increases in frequency with age, and may be greater in lower socioeconomic groups and in high-risk groups such as psychiatric patients. Perhaps 5–15% of the population takes hypnotics at least occasionally and 1–3% use them very frequently. Hypnotic use, like the complaint of sleep disturbance, is more frequent among women and increases with age in both sexes. A relatively small proportion (perhaps one-fifth) of the persons who complain of sleep disturbance consult a physician and fewer still go for the primary purpose of relief from a sleep disturbance. In outpatient practice, hypnotics are most frequently prescribed when the primary diagnosis is a psychiatric or medical disorder, rather than the sleep disorder. Of the total prescriptions written, family practitioners and internists prescribe hypnotics roughly in proportion to the number of office visits they conduct; psychiatrists write disproportionately large numbers of hypnotic prescriptions. The total number of prescriptions for hypnotics in the United States declined 39% between 1971 and 1977, while the number of anxiolytic prescriptions remained relatively constant. There has also been a change in the relative frequency with which various hypnotics are prescribed. The number of barbiturate and most nonbarbiturate hypnotic prescriptions has declined. There has been a rapid increase in the use of flurazepam, which accounts for 53% of all hypnotic prescriptions. Hypnotics are common prescribed to large numbers— perhaps half—of hospitalized patients.

CHAPTER 3

Pharmacology of Prescription Hypnotics

The hypnotics are a class of drugs whose common feature is a subjective effect—relief from a sensation of poor quality or inadequate quantity of sleep. There drugs possess a variety of chemical structures and have been introduced into medicine over many years. They include the chloral derivatives, introduced in the mid-19th century; the barbiturates, first used medically at the beginning of this century; several classes of heterocyclic compounds introduced since the 1950s; and the benzodiazepines, which have had a meteoric rise in use since the 1960s.

Many of these drugs share, to varying degrees, some general properties. Most of them are useful in the treatment of anxiety, and they are often marketed for both anxiolytic and sleep-inducing properties. Many have anticonvulsant properties; in fact, compounds similar to the hypnotic barbiturates and benzodiazepines are employed medically for this purpose. Generally they do not provide analgesia, except in very high doses resulting in profound unconsciousness. In fact, the use of hypnotic doses in patients with pain may sometimes result in undesirable states of excitement. Many of these agents are toxic in overdose and have a potential for the development of physical dependence. A common history in this field is for new drugs to be developed with the claim that they retain potent hypnotic qualities without acute toxicity and potential for dependence; then, with unhappy experience the latter qualities become apparent.

The pharmacology of prescription hypnotics will be reviewed here. Other methods of dealing with insomnia, including over-the-counter hypnotics, L-tryptophan, and ethanol are described in Chapter 10. It may be well, however, first to review briefly some general principles of drug action.

PHARMACOLOGIC CONSIDERATIONS

An important goal in the use of hypnotics is that their effects have a precise duration; it is desirable that they induce and maintain sleep after bedtime, cease acting the next day, and then produce a potent new effect the following evening when administered again at bedtime. (The exception to this would be when it is desired that the drug produce both sleep induction at night and daytime sedation.) As a general principle, the intensity of a drug's effects (therapeutic or toxic) is dependent on its concentration at the site where it acts (Greenblatt & Koch-Weser, 1975). In the case of hypnotics, this translates into the goal of rapidly achieving effective concentrations in the brain at night, with substantially diminished concentrations during the day. If significant amounts of active drug were to remain the next day, unwanted sedation or side effects would be likely to be present; if significant levels are still present the following evening when a new dose is taken, the drug may accumulate in the body until a plateau or "steady state" is achieved.

The desired pattern of intermittent action of hypnotics is, of course, not necessarily appropriate for other types of drugs. Anticoagulants, antibiotics, and antiarrhythmic drugs, for instance, are given with the intention of achieving constant levels around the clock. Since, then, the desired time course varies with different pharmacologic purposes, it is appropriate to consider the factors that determine the onset, duration, and termination of a drug's effects. These include absorption, distribution, metabolism, and excretion. The reader who desires a more detailed discussion is referred to several recent reviews (Breimer, 1977; Fingl & Woodbury, 1975; Greenblatt & Koch-Weser, 1975; Richey, 1975).

Among the qualities of a drug which determine how rapidly it will be absorbed by the gastrointestinal mucosa are: (1) its lipid solubility (the more lipid soluble a drug is, the more freely it will cross the membrane of intestinal cells by "passive transport," the method of absorption of most drugs); and (2) its solubility in the fluids in the gastrointestinal tract (if a drug is insoluble in the fluids in the gastrointestinal tract, it will not be effectively presented to the mucosa). An example of the importance of solubility is found in the various barbiturates; within certain limits, the more lipid-soluble "short acting" barbiturates are not absorbed more rapidly than the less lipid-soluble "slower acting" barbiturates when these drugs are administered as free acids, due to poor solubility in gastrointestinal fluids (Sjögren, Sölvell, & Karlsson, 1965). Unfortunately, the chemical requirements for lipid absorption and solubility in the gastrointestinal fluids are mutually exclusive—lipid solubility and absorption are best when a drug is in its un-ionized or least ionized form (the "pH-partition theory"), and solubility in biologic fluids is best when a drug is in a more ionic form. These seemingly irreconcilable demands are solved by administering drugs as salts, which are water soluble, and which once in solution take on a proportion of ionization related to the surrounding pH. Thus many barbiturates are sold as their sodium salts, a form which is much more readily absorbed by the gastrointestinal tract. Glutethimide is an example of a hypnotic in which poor absorption may lead to a variable time of peak action.

Some properties of the gastrointestinal tract which influence the rate of absorption are gastric motility and blood flow to the intestines. If gastric emptying time is delayed (for instance, by eating a meal just before taking a pill), it will take longer before the medication reaches the small intestine, where the major absorption of most drugs takes place. Decreased intestinal blood flow, such as that which occurs with advancing age, may limit absorption. Under experimental conditions, this effect of blood flow has a relatively greater effect on absorption of the more lipid-soluble drugs, which most easily cross the intestinal mucosa (Winne, 1971); presumably the ability of the blood to carry away the drug becomes a limiting factor with such drugs.

Most drugs are carried to their sites of action and elimination by the blood; although some are simply dissolved in plasma, most are associated to some degree with blood constituents (Koch-Weser & Sellers, 1976). These include erythrocytes and a variety of proteins, but the most important source of binding in the circulation is albumin. It is important to consider the degree of albumin binding for at least two reasons. First, the amount which is bound is not biologically active. Only the free drug is available to cross membranes and hence enter or leave both target and excretory organs. There is a dynamic relationship between the bound and free drug in the blood and the drug in tissues, which may be pictured like this:

$$\text{drug-albumin} \rightleftharpoons \text{free drug} \rightleftharpoons \text{drug in tissue}$$

The affinities of a drug to both albumin and to organ tissues are important factors in the time course and intensity of its action. As the bound and unbound portions of a circulating drug are in equilibrium, the bound fraction serves as a reservoir, releasing more free drug as it is taken up into tissues or excreted. One result of this effect is that albumin binding decreases the intensity of maximum effect of a drug, but increases its duration of action (Koch-Weser & Sellers, 1976). For most psychotropic drugs, those which are relatively more lipid soluble at physiologic pH have a greater affinity for proteins in blood and tissue. The shorter acting barbiturates, for instance, have a higher percentage associated with protein than the less lipid-soluble slow-acting phenobarbital.

A second important aspect of drug binding to albumin is that hypnotics or their metabolites may have such a strong affinity for proteins that they displace other drugs. This is one source of clinical drug interaction. One of the metabolites of chloral hydrate, for instance, may displace oral anticoagulants from protein, causing a temporarily increased anticoagulant effect.

After a drug is in the circulation, its distribution throughout the body is dependent on its physical properties and the degree of blood flow to various tissues. Lipid-soluble drugs rapidly diffuse into well-perfused tissues such as the brain (the "target organ" for hypnotics), liver, and heart, and more slowly enter poorly perfused tissues such as muscle, skin, and fat. This ability rapidly to enter the brain is related to the rapid onset of action of very lipid-soluble ultrashort-acting barbiturates such as thiopental. It also accounts for their rapid termination of activity; as the drug is distributed into poorly perfused tissues, it leaves the brain and blood, and the hypnotic effect declines quickly. This initial period during which blood levels decline due to distribution into tissues is referred to as the "alpha" or "distribution" phase (Figure 13). Although it is part of the profile of the decline in blood levels of all drugs, it is so pronounced as to be clinically important in termination of drug effects only in very specialized circumstances—when extremely lipid-soluble drugs are given by a rapid method of administration such as intravenously or by inhalation. For most drugs the major methods by which action is terminated are biotransformation and excretion. These processes will be discussed in turn.

Biotransformation of most drugs occurs in the microsomes of liver cells, although some agents such as chloral hydrate are metabolized by nonmicrosomal enzymes. Drugs may also be metabolized in other areas such as the kidney and plasma. Very common forms of biotransformation are conjugation of the drug with another substance (often glucuronic acid) or hydroxylation followed by conjugation. These processes may be viewed as having two goals: they may make the drug less active, and they make it less lipid soluble and hence more easily excreted. (The more lipid soluble a compound is, the more easily it is reabsorbed from the renal tubule and hence not excreted; Brodie, 1964.) One of the crucial issues in the evaluation of hypnotics is whether the various metabolites also pos-

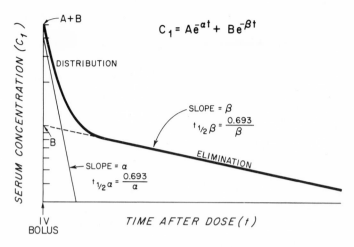

FIGURE 13. Schematic graph of serum concentrations (C_1), plotted on logarithmic scale, versus time (t) after a single intravenous bolus of a drug as predicted by the two-compartment open model. (From Greenblatt & Koch-Weser, 1975, by permission.)

sess hypnotic properties. For the barbiturates and most other common hypnotics, metabolites are relatively inactive. In contrast, in the case of flurazepam and chloral hydrate, the original drug is present in the body relatively briefly, while most of the hypnotic effects are produced by a metabolite which is present for a substantially longer period. The rate of metabolism of a drug is sometimes decreased in the elderly and in various disease states, resulting in prolongation of action of drugs normally inactivated by metabolism. Thus relatively high levels of amobarbital may be present in elderly persons compared to younger subjects (Irvine, Grove, Toseland, & Trounce, 1974). This and other factors such as possible increased sensitivity of the nervous system may result in their enhanced susceptibility to toxic effects (Chapter 9).

In certain circumstances, the rate of a drug's metabolism may be increased because it stimulates the hepatic microsomal system (Breckenridge & Orme, 1971). Hypnotics vary in this quality; the barbiturates are the classic example of drugs that do this, while the benzodiazepines generally do not. This is clinically important because enzyme activation and increased rate of metabolism may be one method by which tolerance (or decreased effectiveness of the same dose when given repeatedly) may occur. This is not always a liability—the incidence of daytime drowsiness does not increase with age (possibly because of enhanced metabolism) when phenobarbital is administered for daytime sedation, whereas this side effect does become more common with advancing years following benzodiazepine administration (Boston Collaborative Drug Surveillance

Program, 1973). Increased enzyme activity due to barbiturates has been employed therapeutically as a treatment for hyperbilirubinemia and kernicterus of the newborn (L. Stern, Khanna, Levy, & Yaffe, 1970; Crigler & Gold, 1969). On the other hand, stimulation of hepatic enzymes by drugs such as barbiturates may enhance the metabolism of other drugs such as anticoagulants and steroids, resulting in their decreased effectiveness.

Excretion of drugs occurs primarily from the kidney into the urine and from the liver into the feces. Other routes include excretion from the lungs, salivary glands, and skin. There may be excretion of the unchanged "parent" molecule or of metabolites. Perhaps half of a dose of phenobarbital, for instance, is excreted unchanged in the urine, while virtually all of secobarbital or pentobarbital is metabolized before excretion. Just as age and disease may influence metabolism, they may alter the ability to excrete drugs (Chapter 9).

Biotransformation and excretion account for the decline in blood concentration during the later "beta" or "elimination" phase of a drug's time course in the body (Figure 13). The rate of elimination may often be described in terms of "half-life," the time in which half of the drug is eliminated from the body. This is possible because most hypnotics are eliminated by first-order kinetics; that is, a constant fraction is eliminated per unit time. This may range, for instance, from a half-life of 5 hr for hexobarbital to 50–100 hr for the major active metabolite of flurazepam. Factors which are related to the half-life include both the clearance (the rate at which the drug is removed by metabolism and excretion) and the volume of distribution (a measure of the extent of the distribution of the drug throughout the various tissues).* It can be seen that the larger the volume of distribution, the longer the half-life, if other factors are held constant. This point will come up later in Chapter 9 because of the suggestion of some authors that increased half-lives of some drugs in the elderly are at least partially due to an increased volume of distribution of lipid-soluble drugs.

If the half-life of a drug is so long that substantial amounts remain when the next dose is taken, the concentration will rise with successive doses until there is a steady state in which the amount ingested is exactly balanced by the amount removed from the body. This steady-state concentration will be approximated (94% of plateau concentration) after

*The clearance (C), half-life during the beta phase ($t_{1/2_B}$), and volume of distribution $V_{d\ (area)}$ are related as follows (Greenblatt & Koch-Weser, 1975):

$$C = \frac{0.693}{t_{1/2_B}} \times V_{d\ (area)}$$

repeated administration over a period of four half-lives of the drug (Figure 14). Although the dose of the drug and the frequency of administration do not influence the *rate* at which a plateau concentration is achieved, they do, of course, influence the magnitude of this concentration. The mean plateau concentration of a drug given once a day can be predicted—it will be 1.44 multiplied by the half-life of the drug (expressed in days) times the peak concentration after one dose (Fingl & Woodbury, 1975). Some of the clinical consequences of accumulation of hypnotics include their daytime residual effects, a subject which has perhaps received too little attention and will be discussed in Chapter 6.

Let us now turn to a general description of the prescription hypnotics and relate these pharmacologic principles to their clinical effects.

BARBITURATES

History

This group of drugs is derived from barbituric acid, a condensation product of malonic acid and urea. There are several different stories relating how Adolph von Baeyer named this compound after synthesizing it in 1864. According to one version he celebrated his discovery on St.

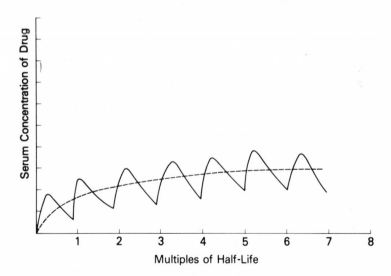

FIGURE 14. Graph of serum concentrations of a drug administered intermittently in a situation in which complete elimination does not occur between doses. Dashed line represents administration of same dose by intravenous infusion.

Barbara's Day, while others have speculated about a barmaid named Barbara (Matthew, 1975). It has been suggested that he considered it the *Schlüsselbart* (the bit of a key), since he suspected it to be the key to a series of compounds (Aviado, 1972). As it turned out, this was an accurate assessment—some 2500 barbiturate derivatives have been synthesized, and pehaps 50 used medically.

Barbituric acid itself does not possess psychoactive properties, which only appear after there are additional groups attached to the number 5 carbon. Diethylbarbituric acid was introduced medically as the first widely used barbiturate hypnotic by Von Mering and Fischer in 1903 (Figure 15). Von Mering had been impressed by the development by Eugen Bauman and Alfred Kast of sulfonal and its ethyl derivatives for use as hypnotics (Leake, 1975). Reasoning that with the sulfonals the addition of ethyl groups increased soporific activity, he explored with chemist Fischer the synthesis of compounds similar to sulfonal, but containing urea and ethyl groups. In the process they condensed diethylmalonic acid with urea. It is said that upon realizing the potential of the drug he had synthesized, Von Mering telegraphed the good news to Fischer, who was then in Verona. According to some stories, Fischer then named it Veronal after the very restful town where he received the good news (Leake, 1975); others believe that the name comes from the Latin *vera*, as he thought it to be the first true hypnotic (Aviado, 1972). Veronal remained the most widely used barbiturate until the introduction by Alfred Hauptmann and others of phenobarbital, or Luminal, in 1912 for the treatment of epilepsy.

During the First World War the blockade of German shipping cut off the supply of a number of drugs which were patented and manufactured in Germany, including Veronal, Novocaine, and Salvarsan (Kogan, 1963). Thus Veronal began to be manufactured in America as Barbital. Interest in this area led to later development in the 1920s and 1930s of short- to intermediate-acting hypnotic barbiturates such as amobarbital, pentobarbital, and secobarbital, and the ultrashort-acting thiobarbiturates used as intravenous anaesthetics. Today perhaps a dozen barbiturate derivatives are in common use.

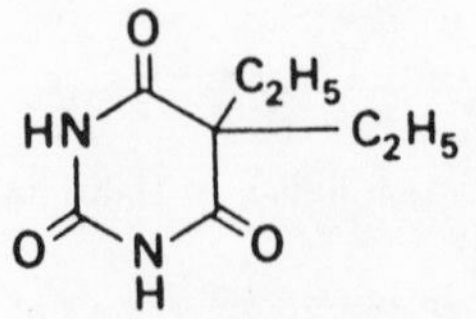

FIGURE 15. Structure of barbital.

Actions

The actions of barbiturates are reviewed by Harvey (1975). They can, of course, induce unconsciousness, either in the form of sleep or surgical anaesthesia, depending on the particular drug, dose, and route of administration. Interestingly, they do not decrease the reaction to pain (and may even increase it in certain circumstances) in doses that do not impair consciousness (Dundee, 1960). All barbiturates inhibit seizure activity in anaesthetic doses; the long-acting agents phenobarbital, mephobarbital, and metharbital seem to have selective anticonvulsant properties which are separable from their sedative effects and are manifest in fully alert subjects. The barbiturates are respiratory depressants, affecting both the neurogenic drive and the responses to hypoxia, carbon dioxide tension, and pH. Unlike the opiates, they have only slight effects on the cough reflex until doses are achieved which have major respiratory effects. Oral hypnotic doses have little effect on the cardiovascular system except for mild decreases in heart rate and blood pressure. Intravenous barbiturates may cause decreased cardiac output, increased peripheral resistance, increased heart rate, or other changes. Barbiturates may decrease gastric secretions as well as the tonus and contractions of the smooth muscle of the gastrointestinal tract, by both central and peripheral mechanisms. They affect renal function both by alterations in renal blood flow (which may be decreased due to hypotension) and direct actions on tubular transport processes such as the sodium and glucose resorptive mechanisms (Blake, 1957). Renal function may also be altered indirectly by barbiturate-induced stimulation of antidiuretic hormone release. In subjects who are not hypersensitive, usual doses do not generally impair liver function significantly. They may, however, competitively inhibit the metabolism of other drugs by cytochrome P-450, and may also cause an increase in activity of microsomal enzymes which metabolize many drugs and endogenous substances.

Structure and Classification

Three sorts of structural additions are made to barbituric acid to produce the medically used barbiturates. As mentioned earlier, substitutions for the hydrogens attached at the number 5 carbon group are necessary for psychoactive properties; these include alkyl or aryl groups in the hypnotic barbiturates and a phenyl group in those with anticonvulsant properties. Sulfur may be substituted for the oxygen attached to the number 2 carbon, thus forming the thiobarbiturates (in contrast to the other barbiturates which are sometimes referred to as oxybarbiturates). A methyl group may be added to the nitrogen at the number 3 position, thus forming the N-methyl barbiturates such as hexobarbital. These latter two groups of barbiturates are used primarily for anaesthesia.

The barbiturates have traditionally been classified by duration of action, largely on the basis of studies of sedation following intravenous infusion into animals (Tatum, 1939). By an extension of such reasoning, agents such as methohexital or thiopental, often used for anaesthesia, have half-lives of 1.5–8 hr (see Table III) and are considered ultrashort acting; those such as secobarbital, amobarbital, and pentobarbital (Figure 16), the group often used as hypnotics, possess half-lives of 14–48 hr and are considered short to intermediate acting; phenobarbital (Figure 17), used for daytime sedation and as an anticonvulsant, has a half-life of 24–96 hr and is classified as long acting. As it turns out, this classification has relatively little usefulness in predicting effectiveness as a hypnotic in acute use. There is actually little difference in patient reports and nurses' ratings of sleep onset, duration of action, and incidence of hangovers among these three groups of barbiturates when given to psychiatric patients for 1 night each (Hinton, 1963). Similarly, medical patients in chronic disease hospitals found little differences in overall efficacy and side effects between 100-mg doses of secobarbital, pentobarbital, and phenobarbital (Lasagna, 1956). The distinction between these groups does bear on some important clinical differences among them, which will be seen in the appropriate sections of this chapter. These include: (1) increasing lipid solubility in the shorter acting agents, which in turn is relevant to the interrelated qualities of distribution, protein binding, and route of excretion; (2) tendency for accumulation in chronic administration; (3) difference in pK_a as a result of which alkalinization of the urine is more effective in enhancing renal elimination of phenobarbital than the faster acting barbiturates (Mark, 1971; see Chapter 5); and (4) tendency to be abused.

Although the barbiturates are not true acids in the sense that they do not contain a carboxyl group, they are acidic and poorly soluble in water (Wade, 1977). They are often pharmaceutically prepared as the sodium salt, which is alkaline, and whose greater solubility in the intestinal tract

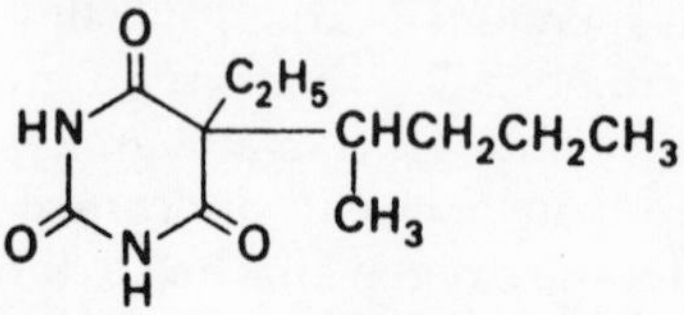

FIGURE 16. Structure of pentobarbital.

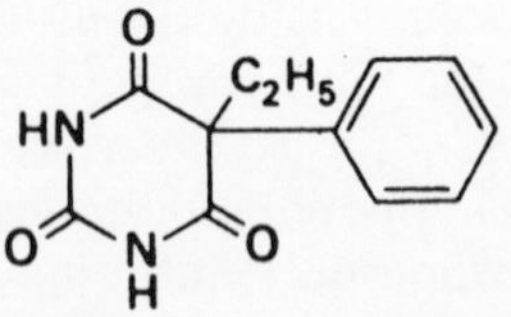

FIGURE 17. Structure of phenobarbital.

TABLE III

Elimination Half-Lives, Apparent Volumes of Distribution and Clearance Values of Barbiturates in Man[a]

Compound	Dose	Route of administration	Mean half-life (h)	Range (h)	No. of subjects	Mean distribution volume (l/kg)	Mean plasma clearance (ml/min)	Reference
Methohexitone	3 mg/kg	i.v.	1.6	1.2–2.1	4	1.13	829	Breimer (1976b)
Hexobarbitone	600 mg or 8 mg/kg	i.v.	4.4	2.7–7.3	14	1.10	259	Breimer, Honhoff, Zilly, Richter, & Van Rossum (1975)
Heptabarbitone	400 mg	oral	4.0	2.6–5.0	5			Breimer & Van Rossum (1973)
	150 mg	oral	7.7	6.2–11.0	7	1.30	138	Breimer & DeBoer (1975)
	6.6 mg/kg	oral	9.7[b]		6			Clifford et al. (1974)
Cyclobarbitone	300 mg/kg	oral	12.0	8–17	6	0.51	35	Breimer & Winten (1976)
Amylobarbitone	3.54 mg/kg	i.v.	22.7±	1.6 (SE)	7 (males)	1.00	37	Balasubramanian, Lukas, Mawer, & Simons (1970)
			20.0±	1.0 (SE)	9 (females)			
	130 mg	oral	24.8	13.7–42.2	10			Kadar et al. (1974)
	120 mg	oral	20.6	16.3–24.3	5			Inaba & Kalow (1975)
	120 mg	oral	23.8	8–40	36		37	Inaba, Tang, Endrenyi, & Kalow (1976)
Vinylbital	125 mg	i.v.	22.8	15–34	28	1.27	38	Endrenyi, Inaba & Kalow (1976)
	150 mg	oral	23.5	19.4–28.8	6	0.79	27	Breimer & DeBoer (1976)
	200 mg	rectal	23.8	17.6–33.5	6	0.88	32	
Quinalbarbitone	3.3 mg/kg	oral	28.9[b]	19–34	6	1.52	53	Clifford et al. (1974)
	100 mg	oral	25.0		6			Breimer (1976a)
	150 mg/70 kg	oral	23.3		6			Dalton, Martz, Rodda, Lemberger & Forney (1976)
Pentobarbitone	50 mg	i.v.	60.3		6			R.B. Smith, Dittert, Griffen, & Doluisio (1973)
	100 mg	i.v.	22.3	14.8–27.7	7	0.99	34	Ehrnebo (1974)
	100 mg	oral	29.6	21–46	10	0.65	20	Breimer (1976a)
	100 mg	oral	26.5	18–48	11	0.80	27	Reidenberg, Lowenthal, Briggs, & Gasparo (1976)
Butobarbitone	200 mg	oral	37.5	34–42	6	0.78	18	Breimer (1976a)

[a] Calculations were based on two-compartment kinetics following intravenous administration of the drugs, and generally on single-compartment kinetics following oral administration assuming complete bioavailability. (From Breimer, 1977, by permission.)
[b] Calculations based on whole blood level data instead of plasma concentrations.

leads to improved absorption. The ultrashort-acting barbiturates are the most lipid soluble, followed by the short- to intermediate- and long-acting agents. As might be expected from their greater lipid solubility, the ultrashort-acting barbiturates enter the brain more rapidly than the other groups; this is, however, a matter of degree, since all barbiturates are readily distributed in all tissues. The rapid entry into well-perfused tissues such as brain is followed by an initial rapid decline in brain and blood concentrations during the redistribution phase, followed by the relatively slower excretion phase. (During the latter, as authors such as Breimer, 1977, have pointed out, many signs of drug effect remain even though anaesthesia has passed.) For the short- to intermediate- and long-acting barbiturates, there is not as clear a clinical difference between the redistribution and excretion phases.

The barbiturates vary somewhat in their patterns of metabolism and excretion. Insofar as the kidneys clear hydrophilic compounds more easily than lipophilic ones, renal excretion of the unmetabolized drug is a significant factor in removal of the long-acting barbiturates (this is true for 27–50% of phenobarbital and 65–90% of barbital). The remainder is excreted in the urine as conjugated hydroxyl compounds. The short- to intermediate-acting barbiturates are mostly metabolized by the liver (also partly by other tissues such as kidney and brain for the thiobarbiturates; Dorfman & Goldbaum, 1947; Gould & Shideman, 1952) and excreted as conjugated hydroxyl compounds in the urine, and to a lesser extent in the feces. Metabolism prior to excretion, most important, involves oxidation of the substituents attached at C-5, but also includes removal of n-alkyl radicals, conversion of thiobarbiturates to their oxygen analogues, and ring cleavage (Nimmo, 1976).

Alterations in Metabolism and Excretion: Illness, Old Age, Enzyme Induction

Blood levels of barbiturates are of course influenced by factors which alter the ability of the liver and kidney to metabolize and excrete them. Among these are decreased functioning related to disease of old age, and increased metabolism related to induction of hepatic enzymes. In the presence of acute or chronic liver disease the elimination of hexobarbital is decreased (Richter, Zilly, & Brachtel, 1972; Zilly, 1974). Patients with acute hepatitis develop sedation sooner during intravenous administration of the drug (Richter et al., 1972) due to a more rapid increase in blood levels (Zilly, Brachtel, & Richter, 1973). This results, perhaps, not only from a decreased metabolism but also from a reduction in the initial distribution space (Breimer, Zilly, & Richter, 1975). Effects of renal failure are complex;

serum concentrations of amobarbital may actually be decreased, possibly due to less protein binding, but concentrations of the major metabolite, hydroxyamobarbital, may be increased due to decreased renal excretion (Balasubramaniam, Mawer, Pohl, & Simons, 1972). Increased cognitive dysfunction occurred in these patients and correlated with concentrations of hydroxyamobarbital; as Breimer (1977) points out, this is a case in which renal failure results in the accumulation of a relatively inactive metabolite, which results in the pharmacological effect observed.

Another group in whom physiologic changes result in altered pharmacological effects is the elderly. As but one example, in the elderly, excretion of 3-hydroxyamobarbital is decreased at 24 and 48 hr after a single oral dose, and plasma concentrations of amobarbital are higher than those of young adults (Irvine *et al.*, 1974). This indicates the decreased hydroxylation (a major form of metabolism) which occurs in the elderly. Coadministration with other drugs may also alter metabolism of barbiturates. Ethanol ingested acutely may decrease the rate of metabolism of a variety of hypnotics, but when taken chronically may lead to increased drug metabolism (Medical Letter, 1974).

Barbiturates administered in repeated doses may stimulate total activity of hepatic microsomal oxidizing enzymes, resulting in increased metabolism of the barbiturates themselves, as well as a variety of other drugs, including oral anticoagulants, tricyclic antidepressants, tetracycline, digitoxin, corticosteroids, and others (Medical Letter, 1977; Parke, 1971). One review listed 49 such drugs whose metabolism might be increased, and hence whose efficacy might be decreased (Parke, 1971). The activity of nonmicrosomal enzymes, such as S-aminolevulinic acid (ALA) synthetase, may also be increased. The increased activity of this particular enzyme may exacerbate the clinical condition of patients with acute intermittent porphyria, in whom regulation of ALA synthetase is already faulty. Other sedative–hypnotics, as well as ethanol, may also induce enzyme activity, leading to increased barbiturate metabolism, a factor in the development of cross-tolerance.

Chronic Administration

When administered daily, barbiturates with relatively long half-lives may be ingested more rapidly than they are eliminated. When phenobarbital, for instance, is given for 22 days, accumulation is evident after the first few days (Svensmark & Buchthal, 1963). In contrast, heptabarbital, with a half-life of 7.6 hr, shows no accumulation after 10 days (Breimer & de Boer, 1975). Relative concentrations of phenobarbital in various tissues after administration for at least a week have been examined in patients undergoing temporal lobectomy due to chronic epilepsy. Concentrations in plasma in such patients correlated significantly with those in brain, cerebrospinal fluid, and skeletal muscle (Houghton, Richens, Toseland, Davidson, & Falcover, 1975); thus sampling plasma concentrations may be a useful indication of brain concentrations. The ratio of brain:blood concentrations has been reported to be 1.13 (Houghton *et al.*, 1975), 0.59 (Vajda, Williams, Davidson, Falconer, & Breckenridge, 1974), and 0.91 (Sherwin, Eisen, & Sokolowski, 1973). Approximately 43% of phenobarbital is unbound in the blood (Houghton *et al.*, 1975). Protein binding to the shorter acting barbiturates is thought to be greater than for phenobarbital (Blacow, 1972).

Tolerance and dependence can result from barbiturate use, and barbiturate abuse is a very real problem of social and medical concern (Chapter 8). Persons who become addicted to barbiturates through recreational use are clearly drawn to the short- to intermediate-acting agents, and much less frequently abuse a long-acting drug such as phenobarbital, presumably due to some difference in the subjective effects. In addition to a potential for inducing dependence, another difficulty with the barbiturates is their marked toxicity in acute overdose (see Chapter 5). It should also be added that there is tentative evidence of an increased incidence of brain tumors in children who were exposed to barbiturates antenatally or later received the drugs themselves (Gold, Gordis, Tonascia, & Szklo, 1978).

The usual hypnotic dose of secobarbital, amobarbital, or pentobarbital is 100 mg.

BENZODIAZEPINES

History

In the mid-1950s, Dr. Leo Sternbach and associates, stimulated by interest in clinical efficacy of tranquilizers, turned to a group of compounds he had examined in the 1930s at the University of Cracow. They had been known since 1891 in the German literature, where they were referred to as 4,5-benzohept-1,2,6-oxdiazines (Auwers & von Meyenburg, 1891). Virtually nothing had been done since the 1930s when Sternbach had studied them. In an interesting series of studies, Sternbach and associates first established that these compounds were not entirely accurately characterized, and in fact had the structure of quinazoline 3-oxides. Having determined that they possessed relatively uninteresting pharmacological properties, they searched for new compounds. When a quinazoline derivative was treated with methylamine, the heterocyclic ring was enlarged to form a product (Sternbach & Reeder, 1961) which demonstrated taming, sedative, and anticonvulsant properties in animals (Randall, Schallek, Heise, Keith, & Bagdon, 1960) and anxiolytic (anxiety-decreasing) actions in humans (Harris, 1960). This new compound, chlordiazepoxide, was followed by the more potent anxiolytic diazepam (Randall, Heise, Schallek, Bagdon, Bauziger, Boris, Moe, & Abrams, 1961), and in 1970 by flurazepam, which was marketed as a hypnotic. Flurazepam and the more recent temazepam are the only bendiazepines specifically recommended as hypnotics in the United States; in Europe and the British Commonwealth, nitrazepam is marketed for this purpose.

Flurazepam

The pharmacology of flurazepam has been reviewed by Greenblatt, Shader, and Koch-Weser (1975), and Greenblatt (1978). In animal studies it shares muscle relaxant and anticonvulsant properties with other benzodiazepines, although less potently than diazepam and very roughly with equipotence to chlordiazepoxide (Greenblatt *et al.*, 1975). In other measures, however, there are some differences. Although a variety of benzodiazepines increase exploratory behavior in mice, flurazepam does not do this (Nolan & Parkes, 1973). A common test of possible anxiolytics is their ability to restore behaviors which had been decreased by noxious stimuli, or reduce behaviors stimulated by noxious stimuli. Although both chlordiazepoxide and flurazepam share the latter property, the doses necessary for such action by flurazepam were close to those which produce motor deficits (Randall, Schallek, Scheckel, Stefko, Banziger, Pool, & Moe, 1969). In the immobilized cat, a variety of benzodiazepines increase high-frequency spontaneous EEG activity, while flurazepam decreases it (Schallek, Lewinson, & Thomas, 1968). Thus, as Greenblatt *et al.* (1975) point out, flurazepam and other benzodiazepines differ in a variety of quantitative and qualitative ways in animal studies, although the clinical importance of these differences is uncertain.

Flurazepam is rapidly absorbed after oral administration, and is distributed relatively evenly in the body. Although diazepam, chlordiazepoxide, and nitrazepam bind to serum albumin rather thoroughly, flurazepam may be relatively weakly bound (Muller & Wollert, 1973). A study in which 28 mg of [^{14}C]-labeled flurazepam was administered to two human subjects indicates that peak concentrations of labeled material appeared 1 hr after ingestion (Schwartz & Postma, 1970). It was only at that time point that the parent compound could be detected, and even that represented only 1% of the total plasma ^{14}C, indicating the rapid metabolism of flurazepam. Approximately half of the labeled material was recovered in the urine in the first 24 hr; after 96 hr, 81% of the label was found in the urine and 8–9% in the feces. The hydroxyethyl metabolite (Figure 18), conjugated to the glucuronide or sulfate, comprised 22–25% of urinary radioactivity. In a study in which spectrophotofluorometric analyses of blood on urine from two volunteers were performed after administration of 90 mg of unlabeled flurazepam, de Silva and Strojny (1971) also found peak levels of the parent compound at 1 hr, but in substantially smaller quantities than the two major metabolites. These included the hydroxyethyl derivative which declined with a half-life of 2 hr, and the pharmacologically active N-1 unsubstituted metabolite which declined much more slowly. After 48 hr, 51–56% of the administered drug could be detected in the urine; over 90% of this material was the conjugated hydroxyethyl metabolite. Kaplan, de Silva, Jack, Alexander, Strojny, Weinfeld, Puglisi, and Weissman (1973) reported on spectrofluorometric analyses of flurazepam in blood following oral administration to four subjects of 30 mg daily for 14 days. The parent compound was present in such small quantities that it was below the sensitivity of the assay (<3–4 ng/ml); the hydroxyethyl metabolite could be detected

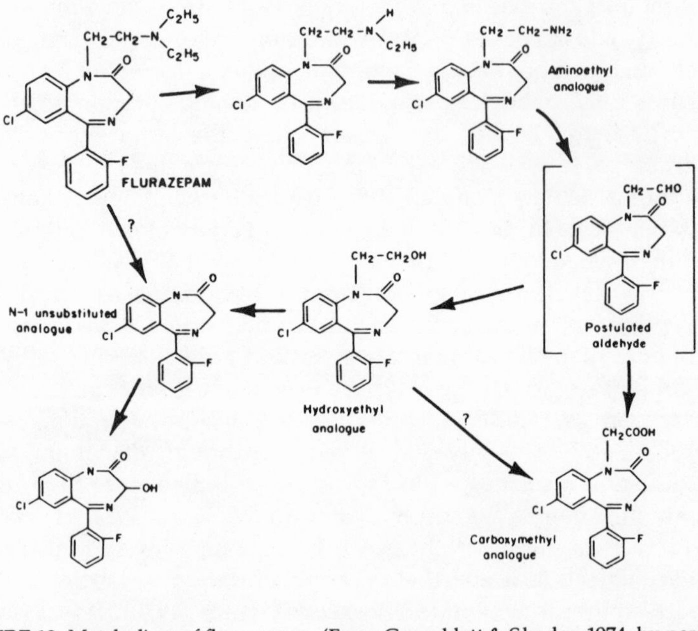

FIGURE 18. Metabolism of flurazepam. (From Greenblatt & Shader, 1974, by permission.)

only in the first few hours after administration. The N-1 unsubstituted metabolite was the major detectable blood metabolite, and had a half-life of 47–100 hr. Over the 14-day period it accumulated in the blood, reaching a plateau in 7 days and achieving concentrations five–six times greater than the 24-hr concentration. As the N-1 unsubstituted analogue shares many pharmacologic properties with its parent flurazepam (Randall & Kappell, 1973), the possibility should be considered that the accumulation of this or similar metabolites might account for the presence of residual daytime effects of flurazepam (see Chapter 6).

Nitrazepam

The pharmacokinetics of nitrazepam have been reviewed by Rieder and Wendt (1973). It is well absorbed (78%), reaching peak blood concentrations within 2 hr. Unlike flurazepam, substantial amounts of the parent compound are detectable in the blood, where it declines with an elimination half-life of roughly 25 hr (range: 21.2–28.1). It is 86–87% bound to circulating protein. Approximately 65–75% can be detected in the urine over 120 hr. Less than 1% of the dose appears as the parent compound; the major metabolites are the 7-acetamido and 7-amino derivatives. There is evidence that nitrazepam crosses the placenta, and small amounts have been found in human milk.

Temazepam

Temazepam is rapidly absorbed. In contrast to flurazepam, only about 8% is metabolized in the first pass through the liver. In tracer studies, radioactivity is found in the blood as a mixture of the parent compound and its O-conjugate. In vitro studies suggest that it is highly (96%) bound to human plasma proteins. It decreases in the blood in a biphasic manner with half-lives of 0.6 and 9 hr, being completely metabolized before excretion. As the half-life of elimination of the metabolites is 2.0 hr, the rate-determining step in its elimination is its metabolism. Most (80–94%) is found in the urine and a lesser amount in the feces (3–13%).

Other Properties of Benzodiazepines

The benzodiazepines appear to have only slight stimulatory effects on the hepatic microsomal enzyme system, and this has not been demonstrated to be clinically significant in man (Harvey, 1975). Other agents which stimulate these enzymes may, however, enhance the metabolism of the benzodiazepines.

Although benzodiazepines enjoy a reputation for producing little respiratory depression, they are not entirely free of such effects. Hypnotic doses of nitrazepam have been reported to produce increases in arterial pCO_2 and decreased central respiratory drive (respiratory response to CO_2) in patients with chronic bronchitis (Rudolf, Geddis, Turner, & Saunders, 1978). Similarly, diazepam employed with endoscopy can produce respiratory depression (Rao, Sherbaniuk, Prosad, Lee, & Sproule, 1973).

In otherwise healthy individuals, acute overdosage of benzodiazepines, including flurazepam, is relatively less toxic in comparison to a variety of other hypnotics (Chapter 5). Mild withdrawal symptoms from benzodiazepines may occur after chronic use of therapeutic doses, and withdrawal psychosis may become manifest up to 14 days after cessation of large doses (Fruensgaard, 1976; "Physical Dependence on Benzodiazepines?", 1977). In general, physical dependence is a much less formidable problem than with many other hypnotics (Chapter 8).

Another potential hazard of benzodiazepines is raised by epidemiologic studies which suggest that use of diazepam in the first trimester of pregnancy may result in a two- to fourfold increase in the occurrence of cleft lip (Safra & Oakley, 1975; Saxen, 1975), although studies with chlordiazepoxide had conflicting results (Hartz, Heinonen, Shapiro, Siskinog, & Sloane, 1975; Miklovich & van den Berg, 1975). Diazepam has also been reported to enter breast milk in sufficient quantities to produce lethargy (Patrick, Tilstone, & Reavey, 1972).

The usual hypnotic dose for flurazepam and temazepam is 30 mg, and for nitrazepam 2.5–10 mg. It is officially recommended that flurazepam be started at 15 mg in elderly or debilitated patients, and this is probably an appropriate caution for temazepam as well.

NONBARBITURATE, NONBENZODIAZEPINE HYPNOTICS

Chloral Hydrate and Derivatives

The introduction of chloroform as an anaesthetic by James Young Simpson in 1847, although met with a variety of medical and even moral criticisms, stimulated interest in the pharmacology of anaesthetics and sedatives. Oscar Liebreich, believing that chloral hydrate (synthesized by Liebig in 1862) would be metabolized to chloroform, speculated that it might have hypnotic properties. Although this rationale was incorrect (it is not converted to chloroform), Liebreich demonstrated in 1869 that chloral hydrate did in fact have powerful hypnotic effects. It has thus become the oldest currently available prescription hypnotic.

Because chloral itself is unstable and not easily prepared pharmaceutically (Harvey, 1975), it was first used as the hydrate (Figure 19). Other preparations include the combination with alcohols rather than water, resulting in chloral alcoholate or chloral betaine. These are broken down in the body to chloral hydrate. Chloral may be combined with phenazone to produce dichloralphenazone. The major metabolite of chloral hydrate, trichloroethanol, has potent hypnotic properties, but like chloral hydrate, it is not conveniently prepared pharmaceutically and produces gastrointestinal irritation. Thus it is prepared as the sodium salt of the phosphate ester, triclofos, which is metabolized in the body to trichloroethanol (Harvey, 1975).

Like barbiturates, chloral hydrate has anticonvulsant effects (although doses necessary for this approach the sedative doses) and has few analgesic properties (Harvey, 1975). Although the dose for anaesthesia is too close to the toxic range to permit use for anaesthesia, a complex adduct with glucose, alpha chloralose, has been used as a laboratory anaesthetic.

Chloral hydrate is rapidly absorbed. Breimer, Ketelaars, and Van Rossum (1974) demonstrated that the parent compound could not be detected in the blood after oral administration, and showed peak levels of the major metabolites, trichloroethanol and its glucuronide conjugate (urocholoralic acid), 20–60 min after administration. The studies of E.K. Marshall and Owens (1954) have indicated that it is in fact trichloroethanol which produces the clinical hypnotic effect. The conversion of chloral hydrate to this metabolite, which may occur in erythrocytes, liver, and other tissues, is mediated by an enzyme important in the metabolism of ethanol. (For discussion of the resultant drug interaction, see Chapter 7.) The blood half-lives of trichloroethanol and trichloroethanolglucuronide are 7.0–9.5 and 5.0–8.0 hr, respectively (Breimer et al., 1974). A small amount of chloral hydrate becomes trichloroacetic acid, which has a half-life of 4 days and which may accumulate during chronic use. Approximately 16–35% of a dose of chloral hydrate is excreted as trichloroethanolglucuronide and 5% as free

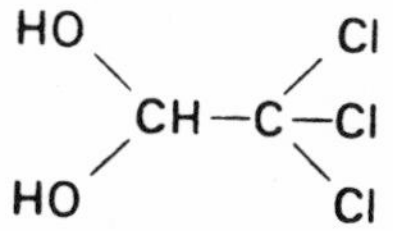

$$\begin{array}{c} \text{HO} \\ \diagdown \\ \quad \quad \text{CH}-\text{C}-\text{Cl} \\ \diagup \quad \quad \diagdown \\ \text{HO} \quad \quad \text{Cl} \end{array} \quad \begin{array}{c} \text{Cl} \\ \diagup \\ \\ \end{array}$$

FIGURE 19. Structure of chloral hydrate.

trichloroethanol (Wade, 1977); a small amount of the glucuronide is excreted in the bile.

Trichloroacetic acid may displace drugs from binding on plasma albumin, possibly resulting in temporary potentiation of such drugs as warfarin (Sellers & Koch-Weser, 1971). Chloral hydrate and trichloroethanol are not themselves metabolized by the hepatic microsomal system, but may in fact stimulate these enzymes and hence the metabolism of other drugs such as dicumarol and warfarin (Cucinell, Oddesky, Weiss, & Dayton, 1966). Thus the complicated possibility that chloral hydrate may increase a drug's action by displacement from binding sites while actually speeding up its metabolic degredation may occur (Harvey, 1975). One can speculate that displacement from binding sites may be a possible mechanism by which chloral hydrate may interact with furosemide to produce potentially serious vasomotor instability (Malach & Berman, 1975).

Chloral hydrate is very toxic in acute overdose, although it occurs fairly infrequently (Chapter 5). Tolerance and physical dependence may develop; in fact, it was actually a popular drug of abuse in the late 19th century. It is extremely unusual today (Chapter 8). Another potential hazard of chloral hydrate is raised by reports that it enters breast milk in quantities sufficient to induce lethargy (Bernstine, Meyer, & Bernstine, 1956).

The usual hypnotic dose of chloral hydrate is 500–1000 mg.

Methaqualone

This drug was first synthesized in an effort to develop a new antimalarial (Figure 20). Its hypnotic properties became apparent and it was marketed in the United States in 1965. Also used as a daytime anxiolytic, it possesses a variety of other activities including anticonvulsant, local anaesthetic, and antihistaminic properties (Harvey, 1975). Oral doses of this 2,3 disubstituted quinazolinone compound are rapidly absorbed. Although the distribution half-life is only about 4–5 hr, the later elimination half-life may be 19.6–41.5 hr (Alvan, Lindgren, Bogentoft, & Ericsson,

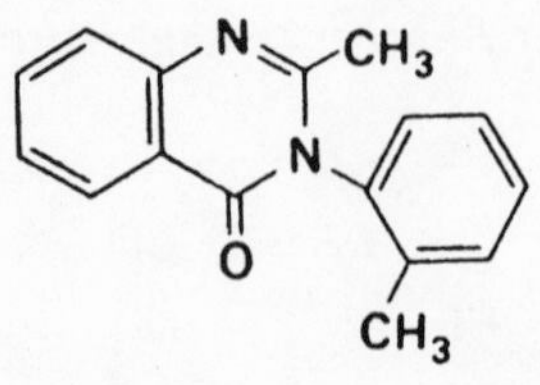

FIGURE 20. Structure of methaqualone.

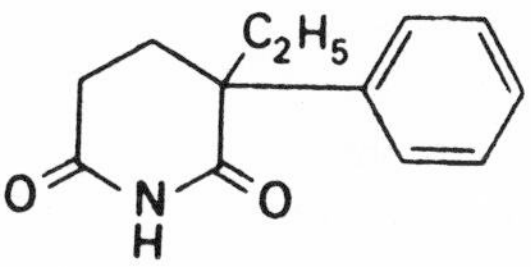

FIGURE 21. Structure of glutethimide.

1973) which may result in accumulation when used repeatedly (Alvan, Ericsson, Levander, & Lindgren, 1974). Approximately 80% is bound to protein (Alvan *et al.*, 1974). It is metabolized in the liver and excreted in the urine and feces; perhaps 2% is excreted unchanged in the urine (Wade, 1977).

Methaqualone, also sold in Europe in a fixed combination with an antihistamine (Mandrax®) has been very popular as a drug of abuse, possibly due to a belief that it provides a particularly pleasant euphoria and that it might possess aphrodisiac qualities. It became evident rapidly that it is very toxic in overdose, especially in combination with ethanol (Chapter 7), and can produce dependence (Chapter 8).

The usual hypnotic dose of methaqualone, N.F., is 150–300 mg; the dose for the hydrochloride is 200–400 mg.

Piperidinedione Derivatives

Glutethimide

Following the introduction of glutethimide in 1954, its use rose rapidly, and it was the most commonly prescribed nonbarbiturate hypnotic until it was superseded by flurazepam in the early 1970s (Figure 21). Later its use declined, perhaps due to the realization of its toxic and dependence-producing properties. It is employed as both a daytime anxiolytic and a hypnotic. It also possesses anticholinergic properties. It is poorly soluble in water, and unevenly absorbed after oral administration. Absorption may actually be enhanced by simultaneous consumption of ethanol, which enhances its solubility. Peak levels are achieved 1–6 hr after administration. Four of six subjects studied by Curry, Riddal, Gordon, Simpson, Binns, Rondel, & McMartin (1971) had an initial rapid decline in blood levels with a half-life of 3.8 hr, followed by a slower elimination phase whose rate was very variable around a mean of 11.6 hr (range: 5.1–22 hr) (cf. Kadar, Inaba, Endrenyi, Johnson, & Kalow, 1974). Plasma binding *in vitro* was 54.2% (Curry *et al.*, 1971). It is mostly hydroxylated and conjugated in the liver; metabolites are excreted in the bile and reabsorbed by the intestine, later to be excreted in the urine as a conjugate or metabolite (less than 2% is excreted unchanged in the urine). This enterohepatic cycle creates particular difficulty in the treatment of overdose (see Chapter 5). Glutethimide administration stimulates the hepatic microsomal enzymes as measured by increased rate of metabolism of several compounds in man, and in animals it stimulates the activity of ALA synthetase.

Methyprylon

Methyprylon, introduced in 1955 and employed as an anxiolytic and hypnotic, is more water soluble than glutethimide. It has a half-life of about 4 hr. Approximately 60% of an oral dose is recovered as metabolites (free or the glucuronide) in the urine, and about 3% of the unchanged drug appears in the urine (Wade, 1977). It has been reported to increase activity of the heptatic microsomal system and ALA synthetase. It may be very toxic in overdose and may produce physical dependence (see Chapters 5 and 8).

The usual hypnotic dose for glutethimide is 250–500 mg, which may be repeated once; for methyprylon it is 200–400 mg.

Ethchlorvynol

This compound is an acetylenic carbinol, a group first shown by Margolin, Perlman, Villani, and McGauch (1951) to have sedative and anticonvulsant effects, which are increased by halogenation (P'an, Gardocki, Harfenist, & Bauley, 1953; Figure 22). It is recommended only as a hypnotic. Ethchlorvynol is rapidly absorbed after oral administration, achieving peak blood levels in about 2 hr (Dawborn, Turner, & Polkson, 1972), and has a half-life of about 6 hr. It is metabolized in the liver and excreted in the urine, where about 10% of the unchanged drug appears (Wade, 1977). It is toxic in overdose and dependence can occur with chronic use (see Chapter 8). Animal studies suggest that ethchlorvynol does not stimulate metabolism of bishydroxycoumadin (Y.C. Martin, 1967).

The usual hypnotic dose of ethchlorvynol is 500–700 mg, and a supplemental dose of 100–200 mg may be given if necessary.

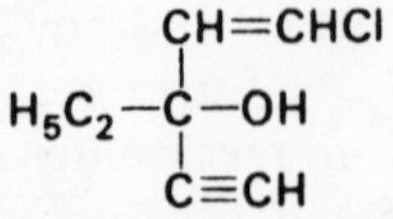

$$CH{=}CHCl$$
$$H_5C_2-\overset{|}{\underset{|}{C}}-OH$$
$$C{\equiv}CH$$

FIGURE 22. Structure of ethchlorvynol.

Ethinamate

Ethinamate is a carbamate, a group which also includes the anxiolytic meprobamate. This hypnotic which was introduced commercially in 1955 is rapidly absorbed from the gastrointestinal tract. Clifford, Cookson, and Wickham (1974) reported that in most subjects there were peak blood levels in 1 hr, and a half-life of 135 min. It is hydroxylated and conjugated in the liver and possibly elsewhere, and the glucuronide is excreted (Murata, 1961). Severe toxicity in acute overdose and the development of dependence have been described.

The usual hypnotic dose of ethinamate is 500–1000 mg.

SUMMARY AND CONCLUSIONS

Hypnotics represent a heterogeneous group of compounds whose common feature is that to some degree they reduce the sensation of unsatisfactory sleep. It should be apparent from this review that no single compound has an unequivocally desirable or undesirable set of pharmacologic properties. Instead, each has its own particular advantages, often counterbalanced by its own disadvantages. One drug may, for instance, be particularly benign in acute overdose, yet have a particularly long half-life which may lead to cumulative effects in chronic use. Another may be remarkably free of side effects when administered appropriately, but the therapeutic dose may be relatively close to the toxic dose range. This raises the possibility that hypnotics with differing combinations of properties might best be used in different clinical situations. Subsequent chapters will relate the pharmacology of the various hypnotics to issues regarding their clinical use.

CHAPTER 4

The Efficacy of Hypnotics

Although there is no shortage of papers on the efficacy of hypnotics, the clinical usefulness of even the most commonly prescribed agents remains unclear. The dilemma is that hypnotics are requested by a vast number of patients, prescribed by many physicians, tested in many laboratories—and yet we have very imperfect understanding of insomnia, which they are supposed to treat. Let us, then, examine some issues in testing hypnotics which result from the elusive nature of the disorder.

In Chapter 1 we dwelt on the difficulties in objectively detecting differences in the sleep of an insomniac. Although the sleep of *groups* of patients differs from noncomplaining controls (in terms of sleep latency, total sleep time, and awakenings) there is so much overlap that one rarely can distinguish an individual insomniac by his sleep alone. Hence the importance of the complaint of poor sleep. The first problem in testing the efficacy of hypnotics, then, is that there are a number of different possible end points. Should a hypnotic be evaluated by its ability to increase the duration of EEG-defined sleep, the subjective sensation of poor sleep, the feeling of well-being the next day, or some other measure? A second problem is that insomnia is not a unitary phenomenon, but results from a variety of disorders (Chapter 1). Just as difficulty urinating may result from a stricture, infection, tumor, or even anxiety, difficulty sleeping may be a consequence of nocturnal myoclonus, sleep apnea, depressive illness, phase lag, and other disorders. (It is not clear how many, if any, insomniacs have "primary insomnia" in which none of these conditions is found.) And just as one would not test a drug for "difficulty urinating" without making a more specific diagnosis, it might be argued that this is just what occurs in many studies in which subjects are selected on the basis of "difficulty sleeping."

METHODOLOGIC CONSIDERATIONS

Possible Measures of Efficacy

There are several methods commonly used to gather data in hypnotic studies. These include:

The Sleep EEG. Among its advantages is the objective and very quantifiable nature of the data. The difficulty is that the clinical meaning of the results is often unclear. In an often-cited study, for instance, A. Kales, Bixler, Scharf, & Kales, (1976) found that 30 mg of flurazepam reduced sleep latency significantly, from 39 to 25.5 min, and total waking time was reduced from 68.8 to 41.7 min. The conclusion drawn from these changes of 13.5 and 27.1 min, respectively, is that flurazepam is of help to the insomniac. What is uncertain, however, is what this change meant in clinical terms—did the subjects experience an improvement in sleep? As discussed in Chapter 1, the relation of subjective and objective measures of sleep is complex and poorly understood. The introduction of a hypnotic further complicates matters. A. Kales, Kales, Bixler, Scharf, and Russek (1976) found that prior to receiving a drug, seven insomniacs (selected by self-report) underestimated their total sleep time; after receiving 0.5 mg triazolam for 1 week, however, they tended to overestimate it (this returned to an underestimation after 2 weeks of drug). Thus it is not at all clear that EEG measures will accurately reflect how the insomniac feels about his sleep. It is also uncertain what the ideal EEG values should be. For instance, it is generally considered a virtue for a hypnotic to decrease intermittent waking time. There is a possibility, however, that a certain amount of intermittent waking is physiologically desirable, and that hypothetical amount is unknown.

Patient Questionnaires. Although these have the potential of reflecting the clinical situation closely, these too have shortcomings. The patient's evaluation may be influenced by nonhypnotic effects of the drug, such as anxiolytic properties, euphoria, or hangover. If the drug produced euphoria, for instance, the patient may give a glowing report for reasons which are less desirable. Subjective reports may also be misleading in the evaluation of hypnotic effects on daytime performance. As will be seen in Chapter 6, patients are often unaware that a particular hypnotic is producing a decrement in performance and in other cases they may believe themselves impaired when in fact they are not.

Measures of Sleep by Other Observers. This is often done by nurses observing the patient periodically throughout the night. Besides the additional complication that the act of observing the patient may disturb his sleep, such reports often relate poorly to EEG measures. Kupfer,

Wyatt, and Snyder (1970), for instance, found that half-hourly nursing observations gave acceptable reflections of EEG sleep time in only 4 of 12 depressed patients. The tendency was to overestimate sleep time. (Interestingly, they were substantially more accurate with schizophrenic patients, presumably because of the patients' bizarre behavior when awake.) A study of medical inpatients with insomnia at a Veterans Administration hospital, however, found a significant correlation between observer ratings and subjective reports of sleep duration and sleep latency (Wang & Stockdale, 1977).

Patient Preference Studies. The advantage here is that there is a clear, easily quantified end point. The difficulty is that patients may prefer one drug to another for reasons not related to effects on sleep. A drug may be disliked, for instance, because of a bad taste or side effects, or it may be preferred because it produces euphoria (a harbinger, perhaps, of increased abuse potential).

Subject Selection

Nicolis and Silvestri (1967) provided a clear demonstration that subject selection could profoundly affect the outcome of a hypnotic study. In an examination of 78 psychiatric patients with sleep disturbance, they found that the administration of placebo or 100 mg phenobarbital resulted in an approximately equal number of observers' reports of "satisfactory sleep" in patients with "mild" insomnia; in contrast, reports following phenobarbital were substantially better than after placebo when patients with "severe" insomnia were examined. The authors concluded that studies will tend to make hypnotics appear more efficacious if the subjects chosen have particularly severe sleep disturbances.

In the years following the Nicolis and Silvestri (1967) study, the problem of patient selection has, if anything, become more complex. With growing recognition of specific disorders which may be associated with insomnia (e.g., sleep apnea), a number of laboratories have attempted to improve standardization by selecting patients who complain of insomnia, are free of diagnosable disorders, and whose complaints of poor sleep are documented by EEG studies. The painful process by which patients are found when these rigorous criteria are employed has been documented by Dement, Carskadon, Mitler, Phillips, and Zarcone (1978), in a report on the efficacy of flurazepam. They found that out of 330 persons who responded to newspaper ads and met the age criteria, only 7 passed the screening procedure and were willing to participate in the study. The advantage of such a process is that the patient group is very well defined and the effects of the drug become easier to understand. The problem, however, is that the patient sample is so carefully selected that it may not be representative of insomniacs as a whole, or of those most likely to take hypnotics. Such an approach also begs the question of how to deal clinically with the person who complains of insomnia, yet has no abnormalities in EEG-defined sleep. (Such persons have been referred to by some sleep researchers as having "pseudo-insomnia," a term they would no doubt resent—the sleep disturbance is very real to them.) A similar paroblem arises in the many studies which attempt to improve uniformity of subjects by using normal volunteers. The price of this particular benefit is uncertainty as to how relevant the data are to the clinical problem.

Another difficulty in subject selection is the tendency to study young healthy adults (volunteers or insomniacs). There are many advantages to this, not the least of which are ease of recruitment and safety. The problem is that these subjects are, once again, not necessarily representative of the population likely to be using the hypnotic in clinical practice. Notably neglected are the elderly, who consume hypnotics in disproportionately large numbers. Some of the complications which result from hypnotic use in the elderly, for whom there has often been inadequate testing, are discussed in Chapter 9.

Other Methodological Issues

Additional considerations raised in other reviews (e.g., Freemon, 1975; Kay, Blackburn, Buckingham, & Karacan, 1976) include:

1. The difficulty of interpreting the effects of a drug unless it is compared to a "standard," a drug in common use whose effects are well characterized.

2. The need for dose-response data. In practice, financial and other limitations usually lead to a single dose being studied.

3. The variable duration of the recording period in different laboratories. One group, for instance, reported that temazepam decreased intermittent waking time (Mitler et al., 1975), whereas another (Bixler, Kales, Soldatos, Scharf, & Kales, 1978) found no effect. One issue in trying to resolve such a difference is that in the former study patients were allowed to sleep until they awakened by themselves, while in the latter they were aroused by the investigators after 8 hr of recording. It seems reasonable to speculate that the method of terminating sleep might also influence the patients' reports of morning sleepiness (Bixler, Kales, Soldatos, Scharf, & Kales, 1978).

4. The possible influence of one night's sleep on the next. Drug-

induced changes in sleep may persist for the next few nights after a drug is discontinued. Hence, it is important to have a "washout period" of several nights between recordings in studies in which drugs are given alternately.

5. The power of placebo effects in sleep studies. Hartmann and Cravens (1973a), for example, demonstrated that administration of a placebo to normal subjects for 28 nights raised the mean amount of REM sleep, and after discontinuation there was a significant increase in both total sleep and REM sleep. A study evaluating the effects of discontinuing a hypnotic might lead to erroneous conclusions unless such effects of placebos—even when they are discontinued—are taken into consideration.

In sum, the results of hypnotic efficacy studies, as well as most clinical investigations, may be profoundly influenced by the methodology employed. What makes this particularly crucial with hypnotic studies is that they involve a disorder which is poorly understood and for which the appropriate measures are not known. These considerations should be kept in mind as we now examine the available data. The studies presented here will be divided into two parts. The first examines the rather sparse literature on the use of hypnotics in specific disorders (e.g., depression, nocturnal myoclonus) which may be associated with insomnia. The second is a reference section which describes the majority of studies, carried out on normal volunteers or insomniacs.

EFFICACY STUDIES IN SPECIFIC DISORDERS

As discussed earlier, one of the major advances in research on insomnia has been the growing recognition that several very specific disorders account for a large percentage of persons who complain of poor sleep. Prominent among these are the sleep apnea syndromes, nocturnal myoclonus, and depressive illness. From this experience one can make the tentative generalization that whenever a disorder producing insomnia is characterized, it becomes clear that hypnotics are not a useful or appropriate treatment for it. More specifically:

1. *The sleep apnea syndromes.* Hypnotics have not been systematically tested with these disorders because of the likelihood that they might further impair respiration, at great risk to the patient. Anecdotal evidence from those performing tracheostomies in patients with obstructive sleep apnea suggests that they are unusually sensitive to respiratory depression from intravenous diazepam.

2. *Nocturnal myoclonus.* It has generally been the clinical experience of investigators that hypnotics are of no benefit in this disorder; systematic evidence is not available.

3. *"Jet lag."* Hypnotics are commonly used for insomnia due to acute time zone changes, although the data bearing on this are sparse and not encouraging. Pollack, McGregor, and Weitzman (1975) observed the effects of 30 mg flurazepam on normal volunteers after acute sleep–wake cycle reversal. Although flurazepam did improve EEG measures of daytime sleep in subjects who had been kept awake all night, they had as much sleepiness the following evening as the nondrug subjects. Allnutt and O'Conner (1971) examined the effects of 5 mg nitrazepam and 100 mg secobarbital on pilot trainees who on alternate nights were put to bed at 8:00 P.M. and awakened at 3:00 A.M. (This study is cited here because their manipulation, designed to test sleep when one arises early, may also be viewed as examining the effects of flying several time zones to the east.) Both drugs decreased sleep latency, and secobarbital increased total sleep time significantly. The subjects reported that they slept better on drug nights, but that in fact when on placebo they had had an "average" night's sleep. On the other hand, administration of either drug did not improve performance tasks the next day, and in one test (signal detection) actually produced a decrement during the afternoon. Subjects often seemed irritable by lunchtime and often apathetic in the evening. There is obviously not enough data from such studies as these to make a very clear statement about the use of hypnotics during acute alterations of the sleep cycle. A tentative implication, however, is that hypnotics may increase the amount of sleep at the new sleep time, but seem unlikely to improve performance or comfort during the new waking cycle. This would seem to reflect the importance not only of the *quantity* of sleep, but *when* it occurs.

4. *Depression.* Although hypnotics are often employed as adjunctive therapy in depression, there are few data on their usefulness. B.R. Ballinger, Presly, Reid, and Stevenson (1974) administered the antidepressants imipramine or desimipramine, alone or in conjunction with amobarbital or nitrazepam, to depressed inpatients. After 3 weeks of treatment there were no significant differences in doctors' or patients' assessments of depression or side effects, or of nurses' assessments of sleep. Similarly, J.A. Smith and Renshaw (1975) compared the combination of the antidepressant doxepin during the day plus flurazepam at night with a daily single dose of doxepin at bedtime in 69 patients with psychoneurotic depression and/or anxiety. Both groups improved—roughly to an equal degree—in terms of depressive symptoms and reports of sleep. The tendency was for greater improvement in the group which did not receive the hypnotic.

A number of studies have been done on groups of psychiatric patients with mixed diagnoses, with variable results. Ananth, Bonheim, Klinger, and Ban (1973) found that 10 mg diazepam, 100 mg secobarbital, or 650 mg chloral hydrate were no more effective than placebo in relieving sleep disturbance of psychiatric inpatients as rated by nurses' and patients' reports. Rickels and Bass (1963), also using nurses' and patients' evaluations, found that several drugs (100 or 200 mg secobarbital, 300 mg methyprylon, 800 mg meprobamate, 500 mg glutethimide) aided the sleep of medical but not psychiatric (schizophrenic or depressed) inpatients. Similarly, Perkins and Hinton (1974) gave 130 and 200 mg amobarbital and 20, 30, and 40 mg chlordiazepoxide on successive nights to 12 neurotic inpatients with anxiety and depressive features. Although EEG total sleep was increased by both drugs, the patients did not perceive the quality of their sleep to be improved. On the other hand, Andersen and Lingjaerde (1969) found that in 26 psychiatric inpatients with mixed diagnoses (22 of whom were considered neurotics), 3 nights of either 5 mg nitrazepam or 100 mg phenobarbital improved sleep on a global patient rating and by nurses' observation of total sleep. Maggini, Murri, and Sacchatti (1969) gave 300 and 680 mg temazepam to eight psychiatric inpatients with neuroses (N = 5) or endogenous depression (N = 3) and found that after 4 and 8 nights there was improvement in sleep latency and total sleep as measured by EEG. The patients experienced the sleep with temazepam as "quieter" and "more refreshing."

In summary, short-term studies of hypnotics in psychiatric inpatients with mixed diagnoses have had variable results. There are very few data on the use of hypnotics as adjunctive therapy in clearly depressed patients, and those which are available suggest that they are of no more benefit than using only antidepressants. Thus the best recommendation at this time is that antidepressants alone are the wisest choice in treating depressive illness with an accompanying sleep disturbance.

REFERENCE SECTION: EFFICACY STUDIES IN NORMAL VOLUNTEERS AND "INSOMNIACS"

Several reviews are available which describe the methodology and results of the vast number of available hypnotic studies (Freemon, 1972; Institute of Medicine, 1979; Kay et al., 1976; Mendelson et al., 1977). This section will summarize the major findings of representative drugs, and deal with the issues raised by these results. Studies on each drug are divided into those employing EEG or non-EEG measures. This is not intended to endorse a rigid division of methodologies (in fact, it is valuable for EEG studies also to include non-EEG measures). Rather, this is a reflection of how a significant proportion of previous studies have been done. Unless otherwise stated, the work presented here meets some basic methodologic criteria (e.g., adequate statistical analysis, use of placebos, at least four subjects) outlined by Kay *et al.* (1976). The material in smaller type is a fairly detailed account of individual studies and is intended for reference; the reader who wishes only more generalized information will find it in the sentences in full-size type at the end of the review of each drug.

Barbiturates

Non-EEG Studies. Pentobarbital is the most commonly prescribed of the barbiturates employed primarily as hypnotics (pentobarbital, secobarbital, amobarbital) and will be considered representative of the group. A number of non-EEG studies suggest that 100 or 200 mg pentobarbital consistently reduces sleep latency and increases total sleep compared to placebo, when administered either for 1 night (Hinton, 1963; Lasagna, 1956; Pattison & Allen, 1972; Teutsch, Mahler, Brown, Forrest, James, & Brown, 1975; Wang & Stockdale, 1977) or up to 2 weeks (Hagenbucher & Kleh, 1962; Sapienza, 1966; Wolff, 1974). Pattison and Allen (1972), studying 50 chronic disease inpatients with reported difficulty sleeping, administered 100 mg pentobarbital, 100 mg secobarbital, 300 mg methyprylon, or 500 mg ethchlorvynol for 1 night each on consecutive nights. Sleep was rated by an observer every half hour. All except ethchlorvynol were different from placebo in various measures (onset and duration of sleep, number of interruptions of sleep), and pentobarbital was most consistently different from placebo. Similarly, Wang and Stockdale (1977) administered placebo followed by 100 mg pentobarbital, 300 mg methyprylon, or 500 mg glutethimide for 1 night each in random order to Veterans Administration hospital inpatients. (It should be noted that in this study the placebo nights used for comparison were actually the washout nights immediately following drug nights.) Nurses' ratings suggested that none of the active medications was significantly more effective than placebo in induction or duration of sleep. The patients themselves indicated that pentobarbital was significantly different from one of the two placebo nights in terms of induction, duration and depth of sleep, but not number of awakenings. On all measures except sleep induction, however, there was a tendency to rate methyprylon higher than pentobarbital. Lasagna (1956) found that in chronic medical inpatients, 100 and 200 mg phenobarbital, 250 and 500 mg methyprylon, 450 and 800 mg meprobamate, 200 mg pentobarbital, and 200 mg secobarbital given for 1 might each were all rated better by patients than placebo in terms of sleep onset, sleep duration, and overall ratings. Sapienza (1966) examined the effects of 2-week treatments with placebo, 150–300 mg methaqualone, and 100–200 mg pentobarbital in a crossover design. Subjects were 50 medical outpatients of whom 18 were thought to have insomnia "without apparent cause." Patient ratings indicated that both drugs were thought to be similar to each other but more effective than placebo in terms of sleep induction, total sleep time, and an overall rating. Hinton (1963) obtained nursing and patient reports after giving a series of barbiturates for 1 night each to 24 psychiatric inpatients (as in the Lasagna study there was no washout period between drugs). Nurses' observations suggested that all barbiturates induced and maintained sleep more effectively than placebo, with the best ratings going to pentobarbital, secobarbital, and phenobarbital. Wolff (1974) assessed the reports of medically healthy subjects, recruited from advertisements, who complained of troubled sleep. One week of 100 mg pentobarbital taken at home was rated by the subjects to reduce sleep onset and wakings and to increase total sleep compared to a placebo. There was, however, no improvement in feeling rested in the morning. Teutsch *et al.* (1975) found that medical and surgical inpatients given 100 mg pentobarbital for 1 night found it more effective than placebo in terms of sleep latency, total sleep, and a global rating. Hagenbucher and Kleh (1962) found that either 100 mg pentobarbital or 300 mg methyprylon, given for 1 week each to elderly chronic disease inpatients, were considered more effective than placebo in terms of a global rating derived from both nurses' observations and patient reports.

Several things should be apparent from the review of these non-EEG studies of pentobarbital. The patients were heterogeneous; most have one quality in common, however, which is that they were in a situation relatively amenable for investigators to study, i.e., medical inpatients or chronic hospital patients. One of the results of this situation is that relatively little information has been gathered about the efficacy in outpatients in medical practice, and no data are available on the subjective experience of taking these very common medicines for more than 2 weeks. This is in many ways illustrative of the data base available in assessing non-EEG effects of most hypnotics.

In summary, at least eight studies suggest that pentobarbital administration for at least 1 week (and in one case 2 weeks) is experienced by subjects as inducing sleep faster and maintaining it longer than placebo. Most of these were done, however, on inpatients with accompanying medical or psychiatric illness, and only two studies document these effects among relatively healthy outpatients.

EEG Studies. Three studies have examined the effectiveness of pentobarbital for 1 or 2 nights in normal volunteers (Baekeland, 1967; Hartmann, 1968) and nondependent opiate addicts (Kay, Jasinski, Eisenstein, & Kelly, 1972). All showed a decrease in sleep latency, and one (Hartmann, 1968) indicated an increase in total sleep. There was a decrease in REM sleep in all three studies, and this was shown to be dose-related by Kay *et al.* (1972). A. Kales, Kales, Bixler, and Scharf (1975) compared 30 mg flurazepam and 100 mg pentobarbital for 28 days in two groups of four subjects each. (Subject selection was based on a history of taking longer than 45 min to fall asleep or of having a total sleep time of less than 6.5 hr.) Waking time after sleep onset and total waking time* were significantly decreased by pentobarbital during the first 3 nights, and during this time there was a nonsignificant decrease in sleep latency. These returned to baseline values by the 12th night.† In contrast, the

---

*This apparently refers to the sum of sleep latency, intermittent waking time (the duration of transient arousals after sleep onset), and early-morning awakening (time from the end of sleep until the recording is terminated).

†It should be pointed out that with the exception of one study containing minimal EEG measures (Ogunremi, Adamson, Brezinova, Hunter, Maclean, Oswald, & Percy-Robb, 1973), there are no data on whether tolerance would be found during long-term use of 200 mg of a hypnotic barbiturate. This seems a crucial question since it could be argued that 200 mg is a more appropriate dose to test in comparison to 30 mg of flurazepam.

total number of waking episodes remained significantly decreased for 28 days. There were small, nonsignificant decreases in percentage of REM sleep in the first 3 weeks of administration. During the initial period of withdrawal, this increased slightly (by 2%), and there was a significant decrease in REM latency.

The data indicate, then, that 100 mg pentobarbital reduces sleep latency consistently when given for a few nights to normal volunteers. A single 4-week study in four insomniacs reported initial decreases in total waking time and number of intermittent waking episodes, but only the latter persisted for the duration of the study. It is not clear whether this evidence of some tolerance by EEG measures is experienced by the patient as a sensation of decreasing efficacy. Nor has it been established how 200 mg pentobarbital would fare in an EEG study of several weeks' duration.

Benzodiazepines

Flurazepam

Non-EEG Studies. Among the many studies which contain non-EEG data on flurazepam, several report on use for 4 days or longer. Reeves (1977) collected sleep questionnaires and doctors' reports from 41 geriatric outpatients who complained of difficulty sleeping and received either 15 mg flurazepam, 0.25 mg triazolam, or placebo for 28 days. Flurazepam was reported to improve sleep onset and quality (but not duration) compared to placebo, with no diminution of effectiveness over the 4 weeks. Triazolam, however, was significantly better than flurazepam in enhancing sleep duration, and tended to be rated higher than flurazepam in all other variables. Viukari, Linnoila, and Aalto (1978) administered 15 mg flurazepam, 60 mg fosazepam, 5 mg nitrazepam, and placebo for 1 week each in a crossover design to 17 geriatric psychiatry patients with dementias or psychoses and who were also receiving neuroleptics. Nurses' ratings suggested a nonsignificant decrease in number of awakenings on the first night and time spent awake on subsequent nights with all drugs. When they were discontinued, there was a significant increase in the number of awakenings with nitrazepam but not the other two drugs. G.W. Vogel et al. (1976), in a study of 12 patients with subjective and objective findings of insomnia, administered 30 mg flurazepam or 0.5 mg triazolam for 4 nights in a crossover design. Questionnaires indicated that both drugs significantly and about equally reduced sleep latency and total waking time. On the 2 nights following discontinuation, subjects reported going to sleep sooner and sleeping more soundly with flurazepam. Dement et al. (1978), in a study with both EEG and non-EEG measures, compared a baseline placebo condition to 28 nights of administration of 30 mg flurazepam. Subjects were seven volunteers with subjective and objective measures of insomnia. Questionnaire reponses indicated a decrease in sleep latency and increase in total sleep time which were significant by analyses of variance but not by the more conservative Greenhouse–Geiser test. Both measures seemed to be returning toward baseline measures in the 4th week. Flurazepam did not significantly affect subjective estimates of arousals. Wang, Stockdale, and Hieb (1975) gave 15 and 30 mg

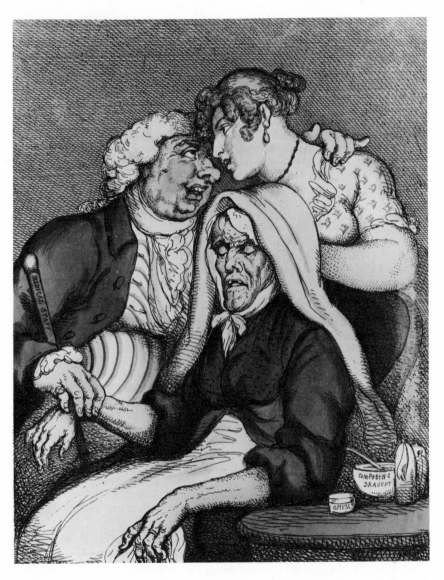

FIGURE 23. This physician seems to have his own particular requirements for hypnotic efficacy. ("Dr. Double-dose," by Thomas Rowlandson, a late 18th-century caricaturist. Courtesy of National Library of Medicine.)

flurazepam, 2 and 4 mg lorazepam, and placebo for 5 nights each in a crossover study of 15 Veterans Administration inpatients with subjective insomnia. Neither dose of flurazepam improved sleep latency as assessed by patient questionnaires. The high dose, however, improved depth and length of sleep in comparison to either placebo or the low dose. In general, both doses of lorazepam were comparable in effectiveness to 30 mg flurazepam. Salkind and Silverstone (1975) reported on questionnaires from general practice outpatients given 1 week's trial of 15 mg or 30 mg flurazepam. Both doses were found to be effective in induction, duration, and overall quality of sleep compared to placebo but did not significantly differ from each other. Pines, Rooney, and Arenillas (1976) found that medical inpatients given 15 mg flurazepam or 100 mg amobarbital (no placebo control) for 1 week rated flurazepam superior in terms of sleep induction and overall quality of sleep. A 1-week comparison of 0.5 mg triazolam and 30 mg flurazepam (with no placebo control) found that medically healthy outpatients rated triazolam more effective in terms of sleep onset and duration, and restfulness in the morning (Fabre, Gross, Pasagajen, & Metzler, 1977). A comparison of 1 week's administration of 0.5 mg triazolam and 30 mg flurazepam in private practice outpatients indicated that they perceived triazolam more useful in terms of duration, depth, and overall effectiveness, while flurazepam was considered more restful (Nair & Schwartz, 1978). Sunshine (1975) administered 15 and 30 mg flurazepam and 0.4 and 0.8 mg triazolam for 5 nights each to medical and surgical inpatients. The lower dose of flurazepam was rated by the patients as more effective than placebo in terms of sleep duration, number of awakenings, and overall effectiveness; the higher dose was effective in these measures and also in sleep induction. The two doses were not significantly different from each other on any variable. Triazolam 0.8 mg was considered more effective than 30 mg flurazepam in sleep induction and duration. Church and Johnson (1979) administered 30 mg flurazepam to 6 poor sleepers with both subjective reports and EEG evidence of disturbed sleep; patient questionnaires indicated an improvement in sleep latency, duration, and quality. Despite these improvements in sleep reports, measures of daytime mood did not improve.

The Boston Collaborative Drug Surveillance Program (1972) reported on the responses of 187 medical inpatients to 30 mg flurazepam, 100 mg secobarbital, or placebo, prescribed for a duration chosen at the discretion of the attending physician. About equal numbers (65 and 61%, respectively) of patients receiving flurazepam or secobarbital considered their overall response to be "good" compared to 43% of those receiving placebo. In a larger study from the same program (Greenblatt, Allen, & Shader, 1977), physicians judged the efficacy of flurazepam in 2542 medical inpatients, many of whom were also receiving anxiolytics. Of those cases in which physicians made a judgment, 85.7% of patients taking 15 mg flurazepam and 91.4% taking 30 mg flurazepam were considered to have a "satisfactory" response.

In sum, two studies indicated that geriatric outpatients and young healthy insomniacs perceived that 30 mg flurazepam was helpful in sleep induction over 28 nights. Several others report such efforts fairly clearly for 1 week. Subjective reports to date have not indicated very much difference between 15 mg and 30 mg in terms of various measures of efficacy. Medical inpatients given 30 mg flurazepam or 100 mg secobarbital at the discretion of their doctors found both drugs to be of roughly equal efficacy in global rating. In a large case series of medical inpatients, most physicians believed it to produce a satisfactory response.

EEG Studies. Reports of 1 (Hartmann, 1968; Johns & Masterton, 1974), 4 (G.W. Vogel *et al.*, 1976) and 5 (J. Kales, Kales, Bixler, & Slye, 1971) nights' administration have suggested the efficacy of flurazepam in increasing total sleep time and reducing sleep latency and intermittent wakefulness. In the 4-night crossover study of G.W. Vogel *et al.* (1976), discussed earlier, both 30 mg flurazepam and 0.5 mg triazolam increased total sleep time and decreased intermittent wakefulness. Both drugs decreased sleep latency, although only the effect of flurazepam reached significance. On the first 2 days of withdrawal, total sleep time after flurazepam remained significantly higher than baseline whereas the values for triazolam were not.

Two studies have examined the effectiveness of flurazepam for 28 nights (Dement *et al.*, 1978; A. Kales, Kales, Bixler, & Scharf, 1975). A. Kales, Kales, Bixler, and Scharf (1975) studied four subjects who reported that they took more than 45 min to fall asleep or slept less than 6.5 hr, and performed sleep studies at intervals over a 3-night baseline period, 28 nights on 30 mg flurazepam, and a 15-day withdrawal period. (As part of the same study, a separate group was given pentobarbital, as discussed earlier.) The duration of the study was held constant at 8 hr. It was found that sleep time rose by 6–8%, and intermittent waking time decreased by 14–17 min over the 28-day period. Sleep latency was decreased significantly only on nights 11–13 in this study. Percentage REM sleep was significantly decreased on drug nights 1–3, 12–13, and 27–28, as was percentage of Stage 3 on nights 1–3 and 27–28. On withdrawal nights 1–3 and 13–15 there was no EEG evidence of decreased sleep or REM rebound. In a later report by A. Kales, Kales, Bixler, and Scharf (1976) which combined the data from other studies, sleep latency was decreased starting on the second night. Similarly, total waking time and intermittent waking time, although decreased somewhat on the first night, decreased substantially more on the second night.

Dement *et al.* (1978) performed a study of similar design with five subjects who had both subjective and EEG evidence of insomnia, and who (unlike the Kales study) were allowed to sleep *ad libitum.* (Subjective reports from this study have been discussed earlier.) It was found that total sleep time after 30 mg flurazepam was significantly increased by roughly 1–2 hr over the 28 nights, but decreases in sleep latency and intermittent waking time did not reach statistical significance. Slow-wave sleep time was decreased starting soon after the beginning of drug administration; REM time decreased starting in the second week. There was no evidence of decreased sleep or REM rebound on withdrawal days 1–3 and 12–14.

Several studies have noted a decrease in Stage 4 sleep induced by flurazepam, a subject examined thoughtfully by I. Feinberg, Fein, Walker, Price, Floyd, and March (1979). Analyzing data from four normal volunteers given 15 mg for 1 night followed by 30 mg for 7 nights, they observed a change in the distribution of Stage 4 sleep on the first night, characterized by an increase during the first nonREM period followed by a decrease in the second cycle. By nights 6–8, total Stage 4 decreased, and it remained decreased on the first 3 withdrawal nights. Frequency analysis indicated that the total number of delta waves over the night was not changed because the decrease in Stage 4 was accompanied by an increase in Stage 2 (which may contain delta activity although it is less dense). The average delta amplitude also decreased by 28%. As in several other studies (Dement *et al.*, 1978; A. Kales, Kales, Bixler, & Scharf, 1975) total REM sleep was decreased, although its time course was somewhat different than for effects on Stage 4. Total REM sleep was significantly decreased starting on the first drug night, and unlike Stage 4, returned to baseline values during the first 3 withdrawal nights.

In summary, EEG studies suggest that in terms of total sleep time and possibly for intermittent waking and sleep latency, 30 mg flurazepam may continue to have effects for up to 28 nights of continuous use. There is some suggestion that maximum hypnotic effects are not achieved until the second night of use. In the two long-term studies available, there was no evidence of sleep disturbance on withdrawal nights 1–3 or 12–15. Two methodologic points should be considered in interpreting these data, however. The uncertainty of the effect on sleep latency may be related to the time at which medication was given. In the Dement study subjects received flurazepam only 5 min before bedtime; the exact time of administration in the Kales study is uncertain. The favorable withdrawal data with flurazepam should also be considered in the light of the methodology of the studies. Recordings during flurazepam withdrawal (Dement *et al.*, 1978; A. Kales, Kales, Bixler, & Scharf, 1975) were made only on nights 1–3 and 12–15. Because of the long half-life of metabolites of flurazepam, it is possible that withdrawal phenomena might only occur several days after discontinuing the drug, and this needs to be examined.

Nitrazepam

Non-EEG Studies. Several studies of 1–7 nights' administration have found that by various measures 5–10 mg nitrazepam was significantly different from placebo, and of roughly equal efficacy to Mandrax®, methyprylon, and various barbiturates (Andersen & Lingjaerde, 1969; Le Riche, Csima, & Dobson, 1966; Matthew, Proudfoot, Aitken, Raeburn, & Wright, 1969; Morgan, Scott, & Joyce, 1970). Viukari *et al.* (1978) found that 7 nights' administration of 5 mg nitrazepam, 15 mg flurazepam, and 60 mg fosazepam produced a nonsignificant reduction in the number of awakenings measured by nurses in psychogeriatric patients. Linnoila and Viukari (1976), however, found that 2 weeks' administration of 10 mg nitrazepam or 25 mg thioridazine to 29 psychogeriatric patients significantly reduced sleep latency as measured by nurses' ratings, but only thioridazine increased sleep duration. Two studies which did not employ placebos found nitrazepam roughly equal to other hypnotics in some measure of effectiveness. General practice outpatients reported that 1 week's treatment with 5 mg nitrazepam was roughly equal to 250 mg glutethimide and 50 mg butabarbital in terms of sleep onset and quality of sleep, and was more effective than glutethimide for improving sleep duration (General Practitioner Research Group, 1965). A comparison of 5 mg nitrazepam and 100 mg amobarbital for 3 nights in inpatients with neuroses or depressive illness reported that nurses and patients rated the two roughly equally in terms of sleep duration (Davies & Levine, 1967).

EEG Studies. A 2-night study of 10 mg nitrazepam in six normal volunteers reported decreased sleep latency, waking time, and REM sleep compared to placebo (Haider & Oswald, 1971). Adam, Adamson, Březinová, Hunter, and Oswald (1976) administered 5 mg nitrazepam nightly for 10 weeks to normal volunteers with a mean age of 57 and found that over the period of treatment total sleep time was increased by about 24 min and intermittent waking was decreased by about 10 min. Slow-wave sleep was decreased, as was REM sleep, although the latter phenomenon was primarily in the first half of the night. During recordings on the first 7 nights of withdrawal, there was a decrease in total sleep and an increase in intermittent waking, but no real rebound increase in REM sleep. This seemed to suggest that nitrazepam might be useful in the long term, although EEG sleep is disturbed substantially during withdrawal.

In sum, a number of non-EEG studies in various patient groups report nitrazepam to be more effective than placebo and usually comparable to other prescription hypnotics in terms of sleep latency and sleep duration. A 10-week EEG study in normal volunteers indicates a small but significant increase in sleep duration and decrease in intermittent wakefulness, but also reports very disturbed sleep upon withdrawal.

Temazepam

Non-EEG Studies. In an uncontrolled study of 147 general practice outpatients who were selected because they "responded satisfactorily" in a 1-week trial, Fowler (1977) found that 133 completed a 12-week course, of whom 90% reported "good" or "very good" benefits. Maggini *et al.* (1969) administered 300 and 680 mg temazepam for 4 nights each to eight psychiatric patients with neuroses or endogenous depression. Patient reports indicated that their sleep was quieter and more restful. Bixler, Kales, Soldatos, Scharf, and Kales (1978) gave 30 mg temazepam for 28 nights to six insomniacs selected on the basis of having both subjective complaints and at least 30 min of EEG total wake time in the laboratory. The only consistent subjective report was decreased number of awakenings. Increased sleepiness in the morning was reported during the first 2 weeks. Mitler *et al.* (1975) gave 30 mg temazepam for 35 nights to seven insomniacs and found an increase in subjective estimation of total sleep, but no change in sleep latency.

EEG Studies. Maggini *et al.* (1969), in the study described above, reported that temazepam decreased sleep latency and increased total EEG sleep. In contrast, Bixler, Kales, Soldatos, Scharf, and Kales (1978), whose study is also previously discussed, found no effects of temazepam on sleep latency, percentage sleep time, or intermittent waking time. The only positive finding was a reduction in total number of waking episodes throughout the study. Mitler *et al.* (1975), who also reported a failure to affect sleep latency, did find a decrease in intermittent waking time and an increase in total sleep. Bixler, Kales, Soldatos, Scharf, and Kales (1978) postulated that the difference may reflect the controlled bedtime (8 hr) in their study, in contrast to the *ad libitum* bedtime in the Mitler study.

In sum, temazepam might seem to have promise as a benzodiazepine hypnotic because of its short half-life, but the small amount of data available in the published literature shows mixed results.

Nonbarbiturate, Nonbenzodiazepine Hypnotics

Chloral Hydrate

Non-EEG Studies. Brown (1970) administered 1000 mg chloral hydrate for 1 night to 50 psychiatric inpatients complaining of insomnia, having first eliminated those who had responded favorably to placebo. Nurses' observations suggested that the chloral hydrate, as well as 500 mg glutethimide and 300 mg methyprylon, were more effective than placebo in increasing total sleep time. Among the three drugs there was a trend for methyprylon to be the most effective, and chloral hydrate to be the least effective, in maintaining sleep. Rickels and Bass (1963) administered seven hypnotics including 100 mg chloral hydrate for 1 night each to 36 medical inpatients complaining of sleep difficulty. Nurses' observations indicated that all drugs were more effective than placebo in inducing sleep and all but ethinamate were more effective in maintaining sleep. Methyprylon (300 mg) was the most effective of all, and significantly more effective than chloral hydrate in both these measures. The patients' overall evaluation was that all drugs except ethinamate and chloral hydrate were better than placebo, and once again methyprylon had the highest score for satisfactory sleep. (When interpreting both this and the Brown, 1970, study, it should be noted that different drugs were given on consecutive days with no washout period in between.) Jick (1967) found that chronic disease patients with complaints of insomnia preferred 1 night with 15 mg flurazepam compared to 1 night with 500 mg chloral hydrate. S.E. Goldstein, Birnbom, Lancee, and Darke (1978), reporting on nurses' observations of geriatric nursing home patients given 15 mg oxazepam, 500 mg chloral hydrate, or 15 mg flurazepam for 6 nights each, found chloral hydrate to be the least effective in controlling number of awakenings. Ananth *et al.* (1973), comparing 1 night each of 10 mg diazepam, 100 mg secobarbital, and 650 mg chloral hydrate in psychiatric inpatients, found that nursing and patient reports could not differentiate active drugs from placebo. Shapiro *et al.* (1969) questioned the physicians of 1618 medical inpatients. Of the 70% who had an opinion, 70.9% thought that chloral hydrate had good overall effectiveness, compared to 13.9% who considered it "fair" and 15.2% who rated it "poor." Hartmann and Cravens (1973c), in a study of eight normal volunteers who received 500 mg chloral hydrate for 28 nights, found that it did not affect the subjects' estimates of the quality of sleep or how they felt in the morning. It did, however, significantly alter relationships between the subjective reports and EEG data in a complex manner.

EEG Studies. Two studies of 1–3 nights' use in normal volunteers showed no significant EEG effects induced by 500–650 mg chloral hydrate (A. Kales, Kales, Scharf, & Tan, 1970; Lehmann & Ban, 1968). Similarly, the chloral derivative triclofos (1000 mg) was without effect when given to normal volunteers for 2 nights (Zung, 1973). A. Kales, Allen, Scharf, and Kales (1970), and A. Kales, Bixler, Kales, and Scharf (1977) administered 1000 mg chloral hydrate for 2 weeks to four insomniacs who reported taking over an hour to fall asleep. Although sleep latency was reduced by 40% during the first 3 nights, this was not statistically significant in the four patients, nor were changes in other sleep parameters. Hartmann and Cravens (1973c), in a study described above, administered 500 mg chloral hydrate to eight normal volunteers for 28 nights; they found that EEG sleep latency was significantly reduced by about 5 min for the first 3 nights, and total sleep time was significantly increased by about 15 min during the entire period of drug administration compared to a comparable placebo period in the same subjects. There were no significant changes in slow-wave or REM sleep.

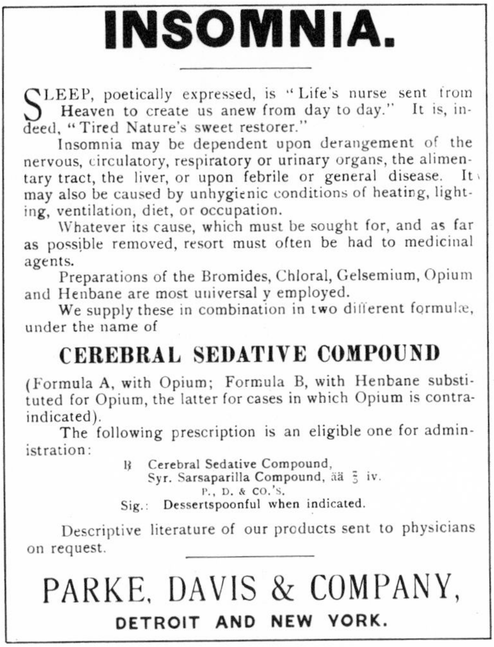

INSOMNIA.

SLEEP, poetically expressed, is "Life's nurse sent from Heaven to create us anew from day to day." It is, indeed, "Tired Nature's sweet restorer."

Insomnia may be dependent upon derangement of the nervous, circulatory, respiratory or urinary organs, the alimentary tract, the liver, or upon febrile or general disease. It may also be caused by unhygienic conditions of heating, lighting, ventilation, diet, or occupation.

Whatever its cause, which must be sought for, and as far as possible removed, resort must often be had to medicinal agents.

Preparations of the Bromides, Chloral, Gelsemium, Opium and Henbane are most universal y employed.

We supply these in combination in two different formulæ, under the name of

CEREBRAL SEDATIVE COMPOUND

(Formula A, with Opium; Formula B, with Henbane substituted for Opium, the latter for cases in which Opium is contraindicated).

The following prescription is an eligible one for administration:

R   Cerebral Sedative Compound,
     Syr. Sarsaparilla Compound, āā ℥ iv.
            P., D. & CO.'S.
     Sig.:   Dessertspoonful when indicated.

Descriptive literature of our products sent to physicians on request.

PARKE, DAVIS & COMPANY,
DETROIT AND NEW YORK.

FIGURE 24. An 1891 advertisement for a hypnotic combination which included chloral, bromides, and opium. (From Hurd, 1891, photograph courtesy of the Library of Congress.)

In summary, non-EEG studies have given chloral hydrate mixed reviews. Seventy-one percent of physicians of medical inpatients believed it to be beneficial in a global rating. Two studies of medical and psychiatric inpatients found it better than placebo in maintaining sleep, but tended to favor methyprylon; in another study, psychiatric inpatients could not distinguish it from placebo. Two studies of chronic disease and geriatric home patients tended to favor flurazepam in a global rating and number of awakenings, respectively. There are relatively few EEG data in insomniacs. One study of four insomniacs indicated a nonsignificant reduction in sleep latency and two normal volunteer studies showed no EEG effects. A 4-week study in normal volunteers suggested a transient decrease in sleep latency and small but lasting effectiveness in increasing total sleep time, although the volunteers reported no change in the subjective quality of their sleep.

Methaqualone

Non-EEG Studies. Three studies of methaqualone have shown mixed results. Bloomfield, Tetreault, Lafreniere, and Bordeleau (1967), in a 1-night crossover study of 40 normal volunteers and 27 psychiatric patients, found that subject questionnaires could not distinguish 150 or 300 mg methaqualone from placebo. In contrast, 200 mg secobarbital was reported to be effective in inducing and prolonging sleep. Sapienza (1966) administered 150–300 mg methaqualone, 100–200 mg pentobarbital, and placebo for 2 weeks each to 50 insomniac outpatients (in 18 of whom there was no clear associated medical or psychiatric condition). Both drugs were found to be of equal efficacy, and significantly more efficacious than placebo in terms of patient reports of sleep induction and duration, and number of awakenings. In an uncontrolled study, Lélek and Danhauser (1970) placed 60 medical and psychiatric patients on 200 mg methaqualone for 8–14 nights. They reported "undisturbed sleep and smooth awakening" in 65%.

Mandrax® (250 mg methaqualone and 25 mg diphenhydramine) has been reported with favorable results in two studies. Haider (1968), in a crossover study in which 48 psychogeriatric patients received 3 nights' each of Mandrax® or 650 mg dichloralphenazone, found that nurses viewed Mandrax® as significantly the more effective of the two in terms of sleep onset and total sleep. Nurses consistently preferred Mandrax® in an overall rating, while patients had only a clear preference (for Mandrax®) in one of the three pairs of nights tested. In a 1-week crossover study of 37 medical and psychiatric patients (of whom 10 had "pure insomnia"), O'Connor and Brodbin (1967) found that patients significantly more often preferred Mandrax® to amobarbital. It should be noted that both of these preference studies did not involve the use of placebo and had no washout period between drugs.

EEG Studies. Three studies of methaqualone for 1–3 nights in normal volunteers (Itil, Saletu, & Marasa, 1974; A. Kales, Kales, Scharf, & Tan, 1970; Risberg, Risberg, Elmquist, & Ingvar, 1975) suggested little change in sleep induction or maintenance; they tended, however, to show a decrease in REM and delta sleep. In a 3-day trial of 300 mg methaqualone with ten insomniacs, L. Goldstein, Graedon, Willard, Goldstein, and Smith (1970) reported decreased sleep latency, intermittent waking, and Stage 4, while Stage 2 was increased. A. Kales *et al.* (1977), in two parallel studies, gave 250 and 400 mg methaqualone for 2 weeks to separate groups of four insomniacs. The only effects noted were decreased intermittent waking time with the lower dose and decreased total waking time after the highest dose during the first three nights of administration.

In sum, there is relatively little systematic non-EEG data to support the use of methaqualone alone. An uncontrolled study of medical and psychiatric patients found that 65% reported undisturbed sleep; in contrast, volunteers and psychiatric patients given methaqualone for 1 night could not distinguish it from placebo. A single 2-week study of insomniacs with and without obvious associated conditions found improvement in sleep onset, duration, and number of awakenings. In two studies, psychogeriatric patients and medical and psychiatric patients preferred Mandrax® (a combination of methaqualone and diphenhydramine) to dichloralphenazone or amobarbital, respectively. Three EEG studies of methaqualone report little or no hypnotic effects during administration for 1–3 nights to normal volunteers; two studies found decreased sleep latency or intermittent waking during the first 3 nights of administration to insomniacs.

Glutethimide

Non-EEG Studies. Glutethimide administration for 1 or 2 nights has been reported to be significantly more effective than placebo on various measures when studied in tuberculosis sanitarium patients (Hohenthal, 1969), medical inpatients (Rickels & Bass, 1963; Wang & Stockdale, 1977), and psychiatric inpatients with neuroses, reactive depression, and anxiety reactions (Brown, 1970). In contrast, a number of studies have found glutethimide indistinguishable from placebo. Mellor and Imlah (1966) gave 500 mg glutethimide for 1 night to elderly dementia patients who also were receiving chlorpromazine; nursing observations suggested that it was no more beneficial for sleep maintenance than placebo. Ban and McGinnis (1962) gave 500 mg glutethimide for 2 nights to chronically hospitalized psychiatric patients, and similarly reported no decrease in sleep latency. Powell and Comer (1973) found it no more effective than placebo, and less effective than 4 mg lorazepam for sleep induction, duration, and other qualities when given for 1 night to preoperative patients. Le Riche and Van Belle (1963), in a 4-night study of chronically hospitalized medical and orthopedic patients, found gluthethimide to be indistinguishable from placebo in altering sleep onset or duration whereas secobarbital and methyprylon produced improvement in these measures. In a study with no placebo control, the General Practitioner Research Group (1965) compared 1 week's administration of 250 mg glutethimide, 5 mg nitrazepam, and 50 mg butabarbital in 66 general practice outpatients complaining of insomnia. Nitrazepam was found to be superior to the other two agents in terms of reported sleep duration; furthermore, there were no statistically significant differences among the three drugs for sleep induction or quality of sleep.

EEG Studies. Two studies have examined the effectiveness of glutethimide for 3 nights. L. Goldstein *et al.* (1970), treating ten insomniacs, found no changes in sleep or waking time, or amounts of Stages 3 or 4 or REM during drug treatment or withdrawal; there was an increase in Stage 2 during drug administration. A. Kales, Preston, Tan, and Allen (1970), treating normal volunteers, found decreased minutes and percentage of REM sleep and increased REM latency and Stage 2, which persisted for the 3-night period of administration. Upon withdrawal there was an increase in percentage REM and Stage 4 sleep. A. Kales, Allen, Scharf, and Kales (1970) administered 500 mg glutethimide to four subjects who complained of taking more than an hour to fall asleep. During a 14-night period of administration, it was found that sleep latency and percentage REM sleep were significantly reduced during nights 1–3 but had nevertheless returned to baseline levels on nights 12–14. REM percentage increased significantly above baseline during the first 4 days of withdrawal.

In summary, there have been a number of non-EEG studies of glutethimide given for 1–2 nights to a variety of different populations, with mixed results. In at least four short-term inpatient studies it was indistinguishable from placebo. Also two EEG studies of 3 nights' administration to normal volunteers and insomniacs reported no significant change in sleep latency or total sleep, and a 14-night study of self-reported insomniacs reported a shortened sleep latency on the first 3 nights only.

Methyprylon

Non-EEG Studies. Several studies have found methyprylon significantly different from placebo and usually equal to (or sometimes more efficacious than) other hypnotics. In two studies of 1 night's administration to chronic disease inpatients, 250–500 mg methyprylon was superior to placebo in terms of sleep onset and duration, although 100 mg pentobarbital (Pattison & Allen, 1972) or 200 mg pentobarbital and 200 mg secobarbital (Lasagna, 1956) produced somewhat better ratings. In a 1-night study of psychiatric patients with insomnia (in whom placebo responders were first excluded), nurses' ratings and subjective reports indicated that 300 mg methyprylon, 500 mg glutethimide, and 1000 mg chloral hydrate produced faster sleep induction and longer total sleep than placebo (Brown, 1970). Among the three hypnotics, methyprylon was the most effective in both measures. In a 1-night crossover study of several hypnotics (300 mg methyprylon, 500 mg glutethimide, 800 mg meprobamate, 1000 mg chloral hydrate, 100 and 200 mg secobarbital, 500 mg ethinamate), medical inpatients with insomnia reported that all drugs except ethinamate were better than placebo in terms of sleep induction and total sleep; methyprylon tended to be given the best scores (Rickels & Bass, 1963). The importance of patient selection in outcome of hypnotic studies is emphasized by the finding that none of the hypnotics tested, including methyprylon, was effective in 20 psychiatric inpatients. Wang and Stockdale (1977) administered 300 mg methyprylon, 100 mg pentobarbital, and 500 mg glutethimide for 1 night each to hospitalized medical patients. Questionnaire data indicated that methyprylon was better than placebo in terms of duration and depth of sleep as well as number of awakenings. (It should be noted that in this study the placebo nights were actually the washout nights immediately following active medication.) In a 4-night study of 200 mg methyprylon, 97 mg secobarbital, and 500 mg glutethimide in chronically hospitalized medical and orthopedic patients, methyprylon and secobarbital were better than placebo in sleep induction and duration, as measured by nursing and patient reports (Le Riche & Van Belle, 1963). In a 1-night study in chronically hospitalized medical and neurologic patterns, nursing reports indicated similar effectiveness of 200 mg methyprylon, 10 mg nitrazepam, and 100 mg secobarbital in duration and quality of sleep (Le Riche *et al.*, 1966). Nursing observations of 70 institutionalized patients indicated that 1 week's treatment of methyprylon or pentobarbital was superior to placebo in a global rating, with somewhat better results from methyprylon (Hagenbacher & Kleh, 1962). In a crossover study in which 300 mg methyprylon and placebo were each given every other night for 1 week to geriatric home patients, staff observations and patient interviews found methyprylon to be superior in sleep induction and duration (Velarde & Harris, 1960). On the other hand, two studies of insomniac outpatients (Linet & Rudzik, 1975) and malignancy inpatients (Lomen & Linet, 1976) reported that 1 night's treatment with 0.5 mg triazolam was more effective than 300 mg methyprylon in duration of sleep and a general sense of having been helped by the medication. (These particular studies had no washout period and did not employ placebos.)

EEG Studies. A. Kales, Preston, Tan, and Allen (1970) administered 300 mg methyprylon for 3 nights to seven normal volunteers. Total sleep time was not reported; REM sleep was reduced on the first night, returned to baseline values on the next 2 nights, and was increased on the first withdrawal night. In an uncontrolled study of pediatric neurology patients, methyprylon at an average dose of 151 mg was useful in inducing sleep prior to daytime clinical EEGs in 80% of 278 cases (Winfield & Hughes, 1957).

In sum, a variety of non-EEG studies indicate that methyprylon is more efficacious than placebo in terms of sleep induction and maintenance, and is often compared favorably with other hypnotics in these parameters. The small amount of EEG data is unclear.

Ethchlorvynol

   Non-EEG Studies. Pattison and Allen (1972), in a study in which several hypnotics were given for 1 night each to 50 mostly elderly chronic hospital inpatients, found 500 mg ethchlorvynol to be no more effective than placebo, while pentobarbital, methyprylon, and secobarbital were different from placebo by several measures. Similarly, Rosenlof and Grissom (1957) found that subjective reports by hospital inpatients indicated little difference between 500 or 1000 mg ethchlorvynol and placebo. There have also been a number of more positive studies. Ban and McGinnis (1962), whose study of 20 hospitalized psychiatric patients has been discussed previously, found that observations and patient questionnaires rated 500 mg ethchlorvynol superior to placebo or 500 mg glutethimide in inducing sleep. Le Riche and Csima (1964), who gave 500 mg ethchlorvynol, 500 mg glutethimide, 500 mg chloral hydrate, and 100 mg secobarbital for 5 nights each to 25 elderly long-term inpatients, reported nurses' ratings showing that all drugs significantly and equally improved length and quality of sleep compared to placebo. Mellor and Imlah (1966) gave 500 mg ethchlorvynol, 500 mg glutethimide, and 200 mg amobarbital for 1 night each to 40 female psychiatric patients with dementia, who were also receiving chlorpromazine. Hourly nurses' observations indicated that ethchlorvynol and amobarbital, but not glutethimide, resulted in increased sleep compared to placebo.
   EEG Studies. In two 14-night studies of four subjects each, 500 mg ethchlorvynol was found to have no effect on sleep latency, intermittent waking time, or total waking time (A. Kales *et al.*, 1977; Kripke, Lavie, & Hernandez, 1978).

In sum, non-EEG studies of ethchlorvynol have been fairly equally divided, and the small amount of EEG data available is rather negative.

SUMMARY AND CONCLUSIONS

Our knowledge of the efficacy of hypnotics is limited by our rudimentary understanding of the nature of insomnia. Thus it is not entirely clear what the appropriate outcome measures in hypnotic studies should be. Each of the commonly used measures—the sleep EEG, patient reports, and nursing observations—has its own advantages and limitations; presumably a complete evaluation of a hypnotic should include a combination of these plus other factors such as evaluations of daytime sleepiness and residual effects on performance. Because of the substantial overlap of insomniacs and noncomplaining subjects in terms of sleep latency and total sleep time, it is not certain who should be studied. Insomniacs with EEG changes in their sleep, for instance, may be desirable because of the objective measure of their disorder, but they are not necessarily representative of those who consume hypnotics. In those cases in which syndromes associated with insomnia are defined, the use of hypnotics is probably of no benefit (nocturnal myoclonus, depression) or potentially harmful (sleep apnea).

In spite of this shortcoming in our understanding, there is a flourishing literature on the efficacy of hypnotics; because of it, the literature is very difficult to interpret meaningfully. Studies of a few nights' duration seem to indicate that most prescription hypnotics affect sleep in some combination of non-EEG or EEG measures. Those which seem to have the least convincing empirical data are glutethimide, ethchlorvynol, and methaqualone. Among those with more substantial efficacy data, there may be differences in rapidity of effect; there is some evidence that agents such as pentobarbital and chloral hydrate reduce sleep latency starting on the first night of administration, while in one extensive study maximal effects of flurazepam did not seem to occur until the second night. The reports of longest continual use indicate small but significant increases in total sleep for 28 nights of chloral hydrate in normal volunteers and flurazepam in insomniacs, and for 10 weeks of nitrazepam in normal volunteers. It is not known if tolerance to EEG effects occurs in long-term treatment with 200 mg of a hypnotic barbiturate. The meaning of these studies will be clearer when further work is done using well-defined insomniac stubjects, combinations of EEG and non-EEG measures, and intermittent as well as nightly administration.

CHAPTER 5

Suicide and Hypnotics

Having reviewed the history, pharmacology, and efficacy of hypnotics, it is appropriate to turn now to the risks associated with their widespread use. Certainly one which has received a great deal of attention has been their use in suicides. (There is a tendency, in fact, to think only of this and dependence as the major negative consequences of hypnotic use, although a variety of problems discussed in later chapters, such as daytime residual effects and drug interactions, should be considered.) It might be well first to consider briefly how suicides with hypnotics fit into overall trends in suicide in the last few years (see Table IV), and to describe the persons most likely to take overdoses. The final portion of this chapter will describe the medical and toxicological aspects of acute poisoning with specific hypnotic agents.

INCIDENCE

There has been a small increase in absolute numbers of suicides from all causes in the United States in the last few years, running from 24,092 in 1971 to 26,832 in 1976 (National Center for Health Statistics).* Drug-related deaths which were considered to be suicides (this comprises about

---

*Data on incidence of completed suicides in this section are derived largely from the National Center for Health Statistics, a federal office which monitors all death certificates in the United States. In evaluating the data, it is important to bear in mind that the categorization of a death as suicide, accidental, or undetermined involves the uncertainties of the medical examiner's clinical judgment, as does the statement that a particular drug was related to the death. When multiple drugs are taken but the medical examiner believed that one of them was the primary cause of death, only that one drug appears in these figures. Another difficulty is that sedatives and hypnotics are not codes per se in suicides; rather, there are categories for barbiturates and for other psychotherapeutic drugs.

TABLE IV. Suicide Attempts in Different

Place and time	Source of data	Annual suicide attempt rate per 100,000	Sex ratio (female/male)
Great Britain			
Edinburgh, Scotland, 1970	One hospital— general practitioners	308 female 221 male	1:4/1
Oxford, England, 1969; 1972–73	One hospital— general practitioners	227 female; 127 male 303 female; 139 male	1:75/1 2/1
Bristol, England, 1972–73	One hospital	645 female (ages 15–29) 334 male (ages 15–29)	2/1
United States			
Papago Reservation, Tucson, Arizona, 1969–71	Reservation health workers	61	1:4/1
East Harlem, New York City, 1971–72	12 hospitals	313 female 232 male (over age 18)	1:5/1
Phoenix, Arizona, 1971–73	All hospital admissions— general practitioners	447 (Indians only)	2:2/1
Miami, Florida, 1972	One hospital	152	1:4/1
Boston, Massachusetts, 1964–72	One hospital	377 (estimated)	2/1 (1964) 1/1 (1972) 1:1/1 (1974)
Australia			
New South Wales, 1967–72	Health Dept. statistics	151 female (ages 20–29)	1:6/1
Traralgon, Victoria, 1970–71	One hospital	125	3/1
Canada			
Yukon, 1970–71	One hospital— general practitioners	325 (ages 20–29)	4/1

Countries: Studies Published since 1971[a]

Major age group	Major method (most common drug used)	Reference
15–25	Self-poisoning	Kennedy, Kreitman, & Ovenstone, 1974
20–29	98% self-poisoning	Bancroft, Skimshire, Reynolds, Simkin, & Smith, 1975
15–35	95% drugs (tranquilizers, antidepressants, hypnotics, analgesics)	Morgan, Burns-Cox, Pocock, & Pottle, 1975
20–25	Drug overdose (44%)	Conrad & Kahn, 1974
18–24 female 25–34 male		Monk & Warchauer, 1974
20–29	(Isoniazid—only drug studied)	Sievers, Cynamon, & Bittker, 1975
Under 35	(Tranquilizers, sedatives)[b]	Petersen & Chambers, 1975
20–29	[b]	O'Brien, 1977
20–29	Analgesics and soporifics	Kraus, 1975
15–24 female	(Diazepam, aspirin, barbiturates)[b]	Bridges-Webb, 1973
20–29	84% ingestion of pills (hypnotics, minor tranquilizers)	Kehoe, & Abbott, 1975

Continued

TABLE IV

Place and time	Source of data	Annual suicide attempt rate per 100,000	Sex ratio (female/male)
Sweden Malmo, 1968–70	One hospital	300 (1968) 400 (1969) 405 (1970)	1:1/1
Israel Jerusalem, 1969–72	Central registry	14 (inpatients only)	1:9/1
Singapore 1971	All hospitals	55	2/1
West Indies Trinidad and Tobago, 1972	One hospital	96	Only women included

[a] From Wexler, Weissman, and Kasl (1978), by permission.
[b] Only drug overdoses included.

38% of all drug-related deaths and is probably an underestimation) accounted for 3330 deaths in 1971 and remained relatively stable at 3002 in 1976. Because there is no specific categorization of hypnotics by the National Center for Health Statistics, it is not clear what percentage of these suicidal drug deaths resulted from their use. Barbiturates, which are classified, have decreased, from 55% of drug suicides in 1971 to 30% in 1976. All psychotherapeutic drugs (primarily tranquilizers and antidepressants) rose from 7% to 15% during this time period. An increase in these agents would then be one factor contributing to the relatively constant drug suicide rate during the period in which barbiturate suicides were decreasing.

It is less easy to determine trends in the incidence of suicide *attempts*. Extensive reviews of the world literature (Weissman, 1974; Wexler, Weissman, & Kasl, 1978) suggest that there has been an increase in the period 1960–1971, and that these high rates (well over 100 per 100,000) have been maintained through 1975 (Table IV). The experience of some individual hospitals is that, in contrast to completed suicides, drug overdose is the most common method of suicide attempt (Wexler *et al.*, 1978). Studies in Oslo (Petersen & Brosstad, 1977) indicate that in the last few years barbiturates have decreased as a source of self-poisoning in patients treated in emergency services, while poisoning with benzodiazepine

(Continued)

Major age group	Major method (most common drug used)	Reference
20–29	(Barbiturates, benzo-diazepines)[b]	
21–30	—	Gershon & Liebowitz, 1975
20–29	Drugs—57% Household detergents—21%	Chia & Tsoi, 1974
15–24	Drugs—56% Household poisons—38%	Burke, 1974

tranquilizers and tricyclic antidepressants has increased. In a study from the Yale–New Haven Hospital emergency room (Wexler *et al.*, 1978), there was some increase in self-poisoning with nonbarbiturate psychotropic drugs, which rose from 18% to 37% in the same period. Nonbarbiturate psychotropic drugs were in fact the most common method of suicide attempt in this series, and were more than twice as common as the nearest contenders (barbiturates, other drugs, and wrist cutting). In an analysis of 385 cases of suicide attempts by self-poisoning in a New York emergency room (Holland, Marrie, Grant, & Plumb, 1975), barbiturates were the most commonly ingested drug, either alone or in combination with other agents, in 29% of the cases. Ethanol alone or in combination was the second most common, followed by over-the-counter drugs. (The interaction of ethanol and hypnotics is discussed in Chapter 7, while over-the-counter hypnotics are described in Chapter 10.)

TRAITS OF THE VICTIM

The evidence suggests that persons who "successfully" commit suicide and those who are treated for nonfatal attempts have differing characteristics. Data for 1976 from the National Center for Health Statistics, for instance, show that the majority of suicide victims (73%) are male. Men were by far more likely to commit suicide with firearms, followed by suffocation (e.g., hanging or drowning) and poisoning (Table V). (Since most suicides are committed by men, this also represents the three most common methods of suicide as a whole.) Women were slightly more likely to commit suicide by use of firearms, followed by poisoning and suffocation. For men, the *rate* of suicides per 100,000 rises to a high level at the 20- to 24-year-old age group, then declines, and later rises dramatically with the age after 50–54 (Figure 25). For females (whose overall rate of suicide is much lower) there is a steady rise until age 50–54, and then, in contrast to men, the rate drops with advancing age after 60. In *absolute* numbers, the highest number of male suicide deaths is at ages 20–30, while for women the peak age is 45–55 (Figure 26).

Perhaps half of suicide victims suffer from depressive illness and one quarter (with some overlap) are alcoholics (Murphy, 1975b, 1977). Suicide is committed less frequently by schizophrenics or patients with organic brain syndrome. The suicide rate per 100,000 was estimated in one case series as 566 for depression, 166 for schizophrenia, 133 for alcoholism, 130 for personality disorder, 119 for neurosis, and 78 for organic brain syndrome (Pokorny, 1964).

TABLE V
Death from Suicide in 1976[a]

Method	Total	Male	Female
Firearms and explosives	14,728	12,128	2,600
Hanging, strangulation, and suffocation	3,689	2,834	855
Poisoning by solid or liquid substance:			
Barbiturates	905	347	558
Psychotherapeutic drugs[b]	448	155	293
Other and unspecified drugs[c]	1,569	569	1,000
Salicylates and congeners	80	25	55
Other substances[d]	674	329	345
Poisoning by gas (e.g., domestic, motor vehicle, and others)	2,468	1,651	817
Jumping from high place	861	548	313
Submersion or drowning	494	270	224
Cutting and piercing instruments	437	317	120
Others	479	320	159

[a] Data provided by the National Center for Health Statistics.
[b] Antidepressants, anxiolytics, and others.
[c] Includes nonbarbiturate hypnotics.
[d] E.g., lye, arsenic, strychine.

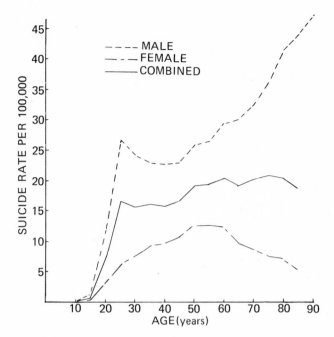

FIGURE 25. Suicide rate per 100,000 population in 1976. Derived from data from the National Center for Health Statistics.

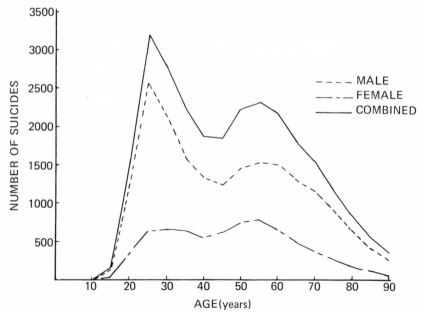

FIGURE 26. Number of suicides in 1976. Derived from data from the National Center for Health Statistics.

Although perhaps two-thirds of suicide victims have a history of suicide attempts or threats, a suicide attempter has only a 10% likelihood of later killing himself (Murphy, 1977). (This 10% figure itself, however, is of course over 50 times more common than the suicide rate of the general population.) The mortality from most overdoses is less than might be expected. In most series there is a mortality of less than 1% among patients who reach the hospital.

CLINICAL TOXICITY

Barbiturates

Overdoses of the various hypnotics produce a generally similar clinical picture, for which barbiturate toxicity is prototypical (P.A. Berger & Tinklenberg, 1977). The degree of severity of intoxication has been classified into several stages by Reed, Driggs, and Foote (1952), and Matthew and Lawson (1966). In the latter, Grade 1 refers to a drowsy patient responsive to verbal commands; at the other extreme is the Grade 4 situation in which an unconscious patient has no response to painful stimulation. Although, as mentioned above, the overall mortality among acute overdose patients who reach the hospital is often less than 1%, Grade 4 coma is associated with mortalities of 5–34% in various series (Winchester, Gelfand, Knepshield, & Schreiner, 1977). Doses of barbiturates associated with fatal outcomes are often in the range of 1.5–2.0 gm.

The clinical findings of toxicity from hypnotics have been described in a number of reviews (P.A. Berger & Tinklenberg, 1977; Dreisbach, 1977; Moeschlin, 1971; Winchester et al., 1977). Mildly intoxicated patients may be drowsy, confused, and ataxic, with good deep tendon reflexes and a clear response to painful stimulation. There may be lateral nystagmus. With progressively greater degrees of toxicity the patient will be asleep but somewhat responsive to painful stimuli. There will be decreased deep tendon reflexes, constricted pupils, loss of corneal reflex, and decreased respiration and blood pressure. Particularly difficult to manage is the middle ground in which a patient is obtunded, but has sufficient gag reflex to make the insertion of an endotracheal tube impossible. In Grade 4 coma, when the patient does not respond to maximum painful stimulation, the respiration is shallow and slow, but at a later stage may be rapid. The pulse is weak and rapid. The pupils may remain constricted but still responsive to light, and in severe cases become unequal or dilated. Deep tendon reflexes are lost, as is the gag reflex. Pulmonary edema may develop, possibly due to hypoxia or in some cases (ethchlorvynol) to direct toxicity to the lungs (Overland & Severinghaus, 1978). The patient may go into shock, either due to a reduction in plasma volume or to a relative hypovolemia with an expanded vascular space (Shubin & Weil, 1965). This may also result in renal failure. The shock or respiratory arrest may lead to death.

If the patient survives the initial toxicity he may be faced with complications resulting from hypoxia such as nervous system damage, renal failure, pneumonia, or pulmonary abscesses acquired while in coma. He may have large blisters of the skin and occasionally may develop ischemic necrosis of a limb due to lying immobile for extended periods before being discovered. A consequent myoglobinuria may also result in renal failure (Moeschlin, 1971).

Benzodiazepines

Overdoses of benzodiazepines are clearly much more benign than those of barbiturates and other nonbarbiturates. Although medical examiner reports in the Drug Abuse Warning Network (DAWN) system list some deaths associated with flurazepam alone, it is not clear that a death has ever been well documented and confirmed with toxicologic analyses. On the other hand, deaths from a combination of nitrazepam (Torry, 1976) or chlordiazepoxide (Rada, Kellner, & Buchanan, 1975) plus ethanol have been well documented. In one series of overdoses, 12 patients were known to have taken benzodiazepines alone, including 2500 mg of chlordiazepoxide and 400 mg of diazepam (Greenblatt *et al.*, 1977). There was little respiratory depression, and only one patient entered Grade 3 coma. Matthew, Roscoe, and Wright (1972), in reviewing 102 cases of nitrazepam overdose, found that none was deeply unconscious, and unconsciousness lasted no longer than 12 hr. In infants, benzodiazepine poisoning may be a more serious problem.

Nonbarbiturate, Nonbenzodiazepine Hypnotics

Overdoses of some of these hypnotics, which are often very toxic, may involve characteristic complications in addition to those already described for barbiturates (Table VI). It can be seen that acute ingestion of approximately 14 doses of most of these agents is likely to have lethal consequences. The physician should be aware of the special qualities of poisoning from some of these.

Chloral Hydrate

Although often considered a particularly benign hypnotic, chloral hydrate can produce severe intoxication in overdose similar to that of

TABLE VI
Fatal Dose and Clinical Findings from Overdoses of Nonbarbiturate,
Nonbenzodiazepine Hypnotics[a]

Drug	Estimated fatal dose (g)	Clinical findings (in addition to those for barbiturates)
Chloral hydrate, triclofos (Triclos)	2	Acute: gastric irritation; rapid circulatory collapse. Chronic: kidney, liver, and heart damage; psychosis; leukopenia.
Ethchlorvynol (Placidyl)	15	Fatigue, headache, confusion, nausea, vomiting, hemolysis, pulmonary edema, acidosis, and pancytopenia.
Ethinamate (Valmid)	15	Thrombocytopenia, liver impairment.
Glutethimide (Doriden)	5	Nausea, pancytopenia, thrombocytopenia, leukopenia, peripheral neuritis, osteomalacia, paresthesia, toxic psychosis, laryngospasm, nystagmus, double vision, pupillary dilation, dry mouth, ileus, cerebellar ataxia, cerebral edema, convulsions.
Methaqualone (Quaalude)	5	Nausea, gastric irritation, vomiting, paresthesia, aplastic anemia, pulmonary edema, convulsions.
Methyprylon (Noludar)	5	Nausea, vomiting, headache, dizziness, possibly leukopenia.
Thalidomide		Neuropathy, fetal injury.

[a] From Dreisbach (1977), by permission.

barbiturates. It is a gastric irritant even in clinical doses, and this may be accentuated in overdose. Acute toxicity may also result in cardiac arrhythmias such as ventricular tachycardia, which has been speculated to result from increased sensitivity of the myocardium to circulating catecholamines (A.J. Marshall, 1977). It has been observed clinically that arrhythmias induced by vasopressor agents are most common after chloral hydrate, barbiturates, and hydantoins (Dreisbach, 1977).

Methaqualone

In severe methaqualone intoxication the clinical picture is similar to that of barbiturates, although hypotension and respiratory depression may be slightly less severe (Matthew *et al.*, 1972). Vomiting and diarrhea are often seen. Pyramidal signs may appear, as may seizures.

Glutethimide

Glutethimide overdoses probably have the highest mortality rate among treated cases of any hypnotic (Arieff & Friedman, 1973; Holland et al., 1975). Particularly worrisome is the fluctuating level of consciousness associated with glutethimide poisoning—the patient may regain consciousness, only later to slip back into coma. This phenomenon has been attributed by various authors to slow release from stores in fatty tissue, poor and delayed absorption from the gastrointestinal tract, and recirculation of the drug in the enterohepatic circulation. Blood concentrations of glutethimide do not relate well to the clinical condition, and there is some reason to think that a better correlation exists with concentrations of a metabolite, 4-hydroxy-2-ethyl-2-phenylglutarimide (Orfanakis & Galloway, 1977). Respiratory depression may be less severe than with barbiturates, but circulatory problems are just as serious. The anticholinergic properties of glutethimide lead to pupillary dilation, paralytic ileus, and decreased bladder function. Matthew et al. (1972), in a review of 1176 cases of poisoning from hypnotics, state that hypotension is particularly a problem with glutethimide. Duration of coma has averaged 48 hr in some series (Maher, Schreiner, & Westervelt, 1962), comparable to values for barbiturates of 40 hr (Setter, Maher, & Schreiner, 1966).

Ethchlorvynol

In addition to the symptomology described above, overdoses of ethchlorvynol by injection have been associated with the development of pulmonary edema (Glauser, Smith, Caldwell, Hoshiko, Dolan, Baer, & Disher, 1976; Rosenthal & Brown, 1976). This has been produced by injection of intravenous ethchlorvynol in dogs, and there is some evidence that the drug produces a direct toxic effect on the alveolar capillary membrane (Glauser et al., 1976). Pulmonary edema is also seen occasionally after overdoses of barbiturates, methaqualone, and other hypnotics. (Overland & Severinghaus, 1978, in a review of noncardiac pulmonary edema, suggested that hypoxia secondary to acute apnea may be the cause of opiate-induced pulmonary edema.) Ethchlorvynol has also been associated with particularly long periods of coma relative to other hypnotics (Matthew et al., 1972), averaging 119 hr in one review of six cases (Teehan, Maher, Carey, Flynn, & Schreiner, 1970). Blood levels of the parent compound correlate poorly with the clinical condition and may be relatively low in severely toxic patients (Westerfield & Blouin, 1977).

TREATMENT

Unlike the situation with narcotic overdoses, there are no generally accepted antidotes to the sedative–hypnotics.* Prior to the 1950s a major goal of treatment of overdose was to attempt to hasten the return to consciousness by the use of analeptics such as caffeine, leptazol, or picrotoxin. Such agents might in fact briefly arouse the patient, although all too often he would relapse into deeper states of unconsciousness. Complications of this treatment also included arrhythmias, hyperthermia, and seizures. During the 1950s it became clearer that conservative supportive measures, often taking advantage of techniques borrowed from anaesthesiology, produced a lower mortality (Loennecken, 1967). This general approach, often referred to as the "Scandinavian method" (Clemmesen & Nilsson, 1961), is to be preferred.

Specific recommendations for treatment of acute toxicity of hypnotics are found in several reviews (P.A. Berger & Tinklenberg, 1977; Dreisbach, 1977; Murphy, 1977; D.E. Smith & Wesson, 1974). In general, the most immediate emergency measures are to assure adequate cardiopulmonary function, then to take steps to remove the intoxicating drug. Other major areas of concern are to preserve good renal function, prevent secondary complications of the comatose state such as pneumonia, and avoid iatrogenic harm (e.g., aspiration pneumonia secondary to induced vomiting, or pulmonary edema due to too vigorous intravenous infusions). Blood gases should be monitored for adequate pO_2 and possible accumulation of CO_2. Moistened oxygen by nasal catheter or mask may be needed, and of course assisted respiration may be necessary. An intravenous line should be started to facilitate administration of medication and fluids. If blood pressure is decreased, plasma or low-molecular-weight dextran may be given while monitoring central venous pressure, which ideally should be 5–8 cm of water. Arieff and Friedman (1972) in a series of 208 overdoses of all drugs except narcotics, reported that giving fluids (usually normal saline) for hypotension was more effective in coma following barbiturate overdoses than with other drugs. Pressor agents may be necessary, although it is well to remember the clinical adage that they are easier to start than to stop (Murphy, 1977), and that they may induce arrhythmias. An indwelling urinary catheter should be used to prevent bladder distention and facilitate monitoring of renal function.

In a conscious patient, emesis should be induced with 15–40 ml of

*There has been a report of rapid return to consciousness of a 34-month-old infant following the use of intravenous physostigmine (H. L. Vogel, 1977), and it will be interesting to see if further work bears this out.

syrup of ipecac followed by several glasses of water, or by 2.5–5.0 mg of intravenous apomorphine. If necessary, excessive vomiting due to the latter can be countered with 0.4 mg intravenous naloxone. (It is thought that emesis is more effective than lavage, as it can also remove some material from the upper small intestine; D.E. Smith & Wesson, 1974.) Emesis is particularly important in the first 2 hr while significant amounts of drug may still be in the stomach; it may be of value for much longer periods of time with some drugs such as glutethimide, which is poorly absorbed and in addition delays gastric emptying. In a comatose patient, emesis should *not* be induced, and an endotracheal tube should be in place (to prevent pulmonary aspiration) before gastric lavage with 10–15 liters of fluid. In the middle ground—a stuporous patient whose gag reflex precludes use of an endotracheal tube—authors such as D.E. Smith and Wesson (1974) recommend careful lavage if the ingestion occurred in the previous 4 hr. They note, however, that in the setting of a major medical center where respiration could be mechanically assisted if necessary, some physicians believe the danger of pulmonary aspiration during lavage to be greater than the hazards of not emptying the stomach. Gastric contents obtained by lavage should be sent to the laboratory for toxicologic analysis. Activated charcoal, 30 gm in 250 ml of water, may then be administered by lavage (Hollister, 1975).

A cathartic such as sodium sulfate may also be given to hasten elimination from the intestines. Castor oil may possibly serve as a ligand as well as a cathartic for lipophilic drugs. (Following up a clinical impression that 500 ml by nasogastric tube every 12 hr reduced the time in coma, Diamond, Brownstone, Erceg, Kieraszewicz, and Keeri-Szanto (1976) reported that in dogs, castor oil every 12 hr reduced the half-life of ethchlorvynol by 13%.) Intravenous fluids (e.g., 5% dextrose in 0.45% NaCl with 20 mEq/l KCl) may be given in amounts of 30–50 ml/kg/day to hasten renal elimination in adults with good cardiac and renal function. Electrolytes should be monitored carefully. Alkalinization of the urine is useful only with long-acting barbiturates such as phenobarbital. (The hypnotic barbiturates are more lipid soluble and hence more easily resorbed; because of their higher pK_a, relatively small amounts will be ionized even at pH 7.7.)

Another method of hastening removal of drugs is by peritoneal dialysis or hemodialysis, which have been reviewed in detail by Winchester *et al.* (1977) In general, these procedures hasten the removal of long-acting drugs substantially and are less effective with short-acting drugs. They are also relatively less effective with drugs which have high protein binding and lipid solubility and poor dialyzability (Gelfand, Winchester, Knepshield, Hanson, Cohan, Stauch, Geoly, Kennedy, & Schreiner,

1977). Another approach which may be particularly useful for more lipid-soluble drugs such as glutethimide, methaqualone, and ethchlorvynol is hemoperfusion. In this approach, which is not in common use in the United States, blood is passed through a filter containing activated charcoal outside the patient's body (DeGroot, Maes, & Van Heyst, 1977; Gelfand *et al.*, 1977; Rosenbaum, Kramer, Raja, Winsten, & Dalal, 1976; Winchester *et al.*, 1977). Originally the method led to problems due to excessive injury to platelets, leukocytes, and red blood cells, and due to charcoal particles embolizing to a variety of tissues, but this was dealt with by coating the charcoal granules with albumin-colodion or polymers. Even with these modifications there may still be a substantial reduction in platelet count, although if carefully monitored it is rarely of clinical significance. Resins such as Amberline XAD-4, which preferentially absorb lipid-soluble organic molecules, may also be used (Rosenbaum *et al.*, (1976). An advantage over hemodialysis is that the equipment is substantially simpler and less expensive. In general, hemodialysis and hemoperfusion are best reserved for severely toxic patients in Grade 4 coma with very high concentrations in the blood.

PREVENTION

The most effective "treatment," of course, is to help *prevent* the overdose. As mentioned earlier, patients with depression are the most common group who commit suicide, and it is important to be aware of the ease with which hypnotics become available to them. The relation of hypnotic use and depression was recently studied by Craig and Van Natta (1978). In a community survey in Maryland, they asked 1830 persons what medications they had received in the past 48 hr, and also administered a depression rating scale. It was found that the two classes of psychoactive drugs which correlated with high depression scores were minor tranquilizers and sedatives. This raises the possibility that these drugs might in some manner predispose one to depressed mood, an issue which has previously been mentioned with reference to benzodiazepines (Hall & Joffe, 1972). Another possibility is that many physicians respond to complaints of anxiety and sleep disturbances in depressed individuals by prescribing tranquilizers or hypnotics instead of antidepressants. There is also reason to believe that physicians are given the opportunity to recognize the illness and intercede in many cases. In one study, about half the victims of suicide by ingestion had seen a physician in the preceding month, and almost one-fourth had done so in the preceding 48 hr (Murphy, 1975a).

SUMMARY AND CONCLUSIONS

There are roughly 25,000 suicides annually in the United States, in which drug ingestion is the third most common method employed. The percentage of these accounted for by barbiturates may be decreasing somewhat, with increases in other classes of drugs. This has resulted in a relatively stable rate of drug-related suicides. Attempted suicides continue at a very high level which may exceed 100 per 100,000, of which drug ingestion may be the most common form. The relative proportions of individual hypnotics among these is not clear, but barbiturates are among the most common single agent. As with completed suicides, there may be an increase in use of benzodiazepine tranquilizers and tricyclic antidepressants. Completed suicides tend to be committed by men over 40 years old who have depressive illness and/or alcoholism; suicide attempters tend to be women under 30 with relatively minor or no psychiatric diagnoses.

Acute ingestion of most hypnotics produces a generally similar clinical picture, which may vary from intoxication not unlike that of ethanol, to coma. Death may ensue from shock or respiratory arrest. Special complications from individual agents included arrhythmias from chloral hydrate, and prolonged coma and pulmonary edema from ethchlorvynol. Glutethimide toxicity may be characterized by a fluctuating level of consciousness related to reabsorption from the enterohepatic circulation or other causes. It produces one of the highest death rates among the hypnotics. Benzodiazepines rarely produce serious intoxication when taken alone but sometimes have been lethal when combined with ethanol. In severe cases when there are high blood concentrations of a hypnotic and the patient is in Grade 4 coma, hemodialysis or hemoperfusion may be employed to hasten removal of drugs from the body. Many of these tragedies can be prevented by early recognition and appropriate treatment of depressive illness.

Residual Daytime Effects of Hypnotics

Among the prices we pay for taking hypnotics is decreased performance on cognitive and motor tasks long after the clinical hypnotic effect has ceased. This problem is compounded by observations that in some cases the patient may be unaware of drug-induced impairment. The background waking EEG and the auditory EEG evoked response may also be altered for many hours on the day following hypnotic administration. Although the significance of these electrophysiologic changes is unclear, they do suggest at least that hypnotics alter normal physiology for prolonged periods, and they are perhaps the most sensitive available measures of residual effects. This section will describe these residual effects of hypnotics on electrophysiology and psychomotor performance, with emphasis on effects which occur at least 8 hr after nocturnal drug administration.

ELECTROPHYSIOLOGIC RESIDUAL EFFECTS

The residual effects on the human waking EEG are usually reported as the mean rectified voltage in each of four or five frequency ranges (approximately 2.4–4.0, 4.0–7.5, 7.5–13.5, 13.5–26.0, and 26.0–35Hz), sometimes presented as an absolute value and sometimes as a percentage of the mean voltage in the whole EEG spectrum. In general, studies on the day after taking either barbiturates or benzodiazepines the previous bedtime tend to report decreased voltage in the slower frequencies of

TABLE VII. Residual Effects

Author	Drug	Dose	Frequency band (Hz)	
			2.4–4.0	4.0–7.5
Bond & Lader, 1975	flunitrazepam	2 mg	↓	↓
Veldkamp, Straw, Metzler, & Demissianos, 1974	triazolam	0.5 mg 1.0 mg	↓[a]	↓[a]
	flurazepam	30 mg	0	0
Malpas et al., 1970	nitrazepam	5 & 10 mg	increased drowsiness and decreased sleep latency at high dose (defined by clinical EEG)	
	amobarbital	100 & 200 mg	no change in drowsiness or sleep latency	
Bond & Lader, 1972	nitrazepam	5 & 10 mg	↓	↓
	butabarbital	100 & 200 mg	↓ high dose	0
Bond & Lader, 1973	flurazepam	15 or 30 mg	↓	↓
	butabarbital	150 mg	↓	0

[a] Used single low-frequency band of 0–7.5 Hz.
[b] DSST = digit–symbol substitution test.

2.4–4.0 Hz, and possibly 4.0–7.5 Hz (see Table VII). The barbiturates, and sometimes benzodiazepines, increase the voltage in the 13.5- to 26.0-Hz range. The 7.5- to 13.5-Hz range has shown either no change or decreases with benzodiazepines and apparently has nonsignificant tendencies to increase with barbiturates. In another approach, visual scoring of the EEG suggested that 18 hr after normal subjects receive 5 or 15 mg of nitrazepam (but not 100 or 200 mg of amobarbital) they are more likely to fall asleep than after taking placebo (Malpas, Rowen, Joyce, & Scott, 1970). Perhaps more germane than the details of these frequency shifts

of Hypnotics on the Waking EEG

7.5–13.5	13.5–26.0	25–35	Duration of EEG effect	Comments on duration of psychomotor testing
0	' ↑	—	up to 18 hr	↓ tapping rate, ↓ card sorting, ↓ symbol copying at 12 hr (not tested at 18 hr).
0	0	↑ high dose	16.5 hr	Card sorting still ↓ at 16 hr, DSST still ↓ with high dose at 16 hr.[b]
0	0	↑	16.5 hr	Card sorting returned to normal after 10 hr—no change in DSST even at 10 hr.[b]
			18 hr	↓ card sorting at 13 hr but not 17 hr.
			18 hr	No ↓ card sorting.
↓	0	—	high dose 12 hr	↑ reaction time, ↓ tapping, ↓ card sorting (motor) at higher dose at 12 hr.
0	↑ high dose	—	12 hr	↑ reaction time, ↓ tapping, ↓ card sorting (motor) at higher dose at 12 hr.
↓	0	—	18 hr	For both drugs reaction time returned to normal by 18 hr. For flurazepam DSST ↓ at 12 hr only. ↓ symbol copying 12–18 hr.
0	↑	—	18 hr	↓ DSST at 12 hr only.[b]

and results of visual scoring is the general observation that changes in the EEG can occur for prolonged periods after the administration of hypnotics, in some cases up to 18 hr (whether they last longer than this is unknown, as recordings beyond this time point are not available). In the majority of those studies in which psychomotor testing was also performed, these tests had returned to normal while EEG effects were still present. Thus the EEG would appear to be a very sensitive indicator of altered nervous system physiology, although of course the practical significance of the frequency analysis data is not clear.

PSYCHOMOTOR MEASURES OF RESIDUAL EFFECTS

A number of studies have reported on psychomotor testing in the daytime following nocturnal hypnotic administration. Table VIII summarizes those in which medication was given at bedtime, and certain minimal methodologic criteria (more than four subjects in each drug group, use of matched placebo groups) were met. Most of these studies tend to use the same group of tests, which include:

Tapping Rate: The subject is requested to tap his fingers on a key as rapidly as possible. This is a test of motor function, derived from the Halstead–Reitan battery for organic brain damage. It is thought to be particularly sensitive to dysfunction of the cortical motor strip.

Simple Auditory Reaction Time. The subject must push a button as soon as possible when he hears a tone. Auditory responses have long been used as a measure of brain damage. Auditory measures which require more discrimination are thought to be particularly sensitive to pathology of the temporal lobe.

Complex Visual Reaction Time. The subject is shown a row of lights and is instructed to push the button corresponding to the particular light which comes on. This is thought to be a basic test of perceptual discrimination, employing relatively little cognitive function.

Card Sorting. The subject is instructed to sort a deck of cards into two, four, six, or eight piles. This test is often performed in two parts: (1) the subject makes several piles from a deck of identical cards, a task which is thought to measure motor function, and (2) he is then asked to sort cards into several piles as determined by symbols which appear on them. The time for the first sorting is subtracted from the time for the category sorting, and this remaining value is thought to be a measure of cognitive function. In some senses this is also a variation on the complex visual reaction time task.

Digit–Symbol Substitution Test. In this test, derived from the Wechsler Adult Intelligence Scale, the subjects are given a coding task in which symbols are substituted for numbers. Sometimes, in a manner analogous to the card-sorting test, a symbol-copying test is also performed in order to parse out the motor component. Vigilance, learning, and coordination seem to play a role, and in some senses this, too, is a form of complex visual reaction time.

Adaptive Tracking Tests. The subject must keep a marker inside a moving track or circle, by use of a steering wheel or joystick, in this test of coordination. The speed of the moving track may either be fixed or may be changed by the subject.

Divided Attention Test. In front of a subject are a row of four dials, two in the center of his visual field and two more peripherally. Each dial, on which there is a revolving pointer, has several marks on its face. Every time the pointer crosses a mark the subject must push a button.

These tests are useful insofar as they are easily performed and provide simple quantified data. It is important to bear in mind, however, that they are somewhat nonspecific, and at best they provide no more than a hint about specific brain functions altered by drugs. It is perhaps more prudent to think of them as useful markers of time-related effects on nervous system function, rather than to make too much of the specific effects produced. Another caveat in the interpretation of the studies summarized here is that specific comparisons among drugs should be made with caution because of the widely differing doses employed. One study, for instance (Saario & Linnoila, 1976), compared 30 mg of flurazepam with 100 mg amobarbital, while in another (Borland & Nicholson, 1975) 200 mg of the barbituate pentobarbital was apparently considered the comparable dose. Thus, comparisons among studies are difficult.

The bulk of the performance studies have been done with benzodiazepines and barbiturates, although such agents as glutethimide (Saario & Linnoila, 1976) and methaqualone (Saario & Linnoila, 1976) have been examined. In general, drug effects have been more pronounced on electrophysiologic measures and mood scales than on objective measures of performance (Bond & Lader, 1973). Still, virtually all of these hypnotics have influenced the various measures, with durations of effects up to about 34 hr in some cases. No single drug or class of drugs seems substantially less likely to produce these residual effects. Some generalizations can be made about these studies, however. First of all, with some benzodiazepines changes may be absent on the first day, yet may appear after taking these agents for a week (Tansella, Zimmermann-Tansella, & Lader, 1974). (This may reflect accumulation of psychoactive metabolites, as discussed in Chapter 3.) Thus, inferences from studies which examine a single dose should not be generalized to what might happen to patients on chronic medication. Another point is that these drugs do not necessarily decrease performance. Administration of diazepam (5 mg t.i.d. for 2 weeks) may actually result in improved reaction times in the choice reaction test (Linnoila, Saario, & Maki, 1974), possibly due to relaxing the subject. On the other hand, these improvements are not usually across the board. In another report from the same group, chronic diazepam administration again improved reaction time and slightly improved coordination in a stimulated driving procedure at a fixed speed, but provoked the subjects to drive faster and make more mistakes when the subjects themselves could set the speed (Linnoila, Saario, & Mattila,

TABLE VIII. Residual Effects of

Author(s)	Drug	Dose	No. of nights of administration	Time of testing (hr after last dose)	Simple auditory reaction time	Complex visual reaction time [b]
				Test[a]		
Bond & Lader, 1973	butabarbital	150 mg	1	12, 15, 18	0	0
	flurazepam	15, 30 mg	1	12, 15, 18	0	0
Bond & Lader, 1972	butabarbital	100, 200 mg	1	12	↓[c]	
	nitrazepam	5, 10 mg	1	12	↓[c]	
Bond & Lader, 1975	flunitrazepam	1, 2 mg	1	12	0	
Borland & Nicholson, 1975	nitrazepam	10 mg	1	10–34		↓34 hr
	flurazepam	30 mg	1	10–34		↓16 hr
	pentobarbital	200 mg	1	10–34		↓34 hr
Malpas et al., 1970	nitrazepam	5, 10 mg	1	13–17		
	amobarbital	100, 200 mg	1	13–17		
Veldkamp et al., 1974	triazolam	0.5, 1.0 mg	1	10–16		
	flurazepam	30 mg	1	10–16		
Saario & Linnoila, 1976	amobarbital	100 mg	7	10.5–13		0[e]
	flurazepam	30 mg	7	10.5–13		0[e]
	methaqualone-diphenhydramine	250/25mg	14	10.5–13		0[e]
	glutethimide	250 mg	14	10.5–13		0[e]
Tansella et al., 1974[d]	N-desmethyl-diazepam	10, 20 mg	1 & 7	11	0	
	amobarbital	200 mg	1 & 7	11	0	
Saario, Linnoila, & Maki, 1975	morphanthridine	10 mg	14	10.5–13		0
	nitrazepam	10 mg	14	10.5–13		0
Hindmarch, Parrott, & Arerillas, 1977	flunitrazepam	1 mg	2 + 4	~9.5–12		0
	amobarbital	100 mg	2 + 4	~9.5–12		0
	dichloral-phenazone	1300 mg	2 + 4	9.5–12		0[b]
McKenzie & Elliott, 1965	secobarbital	200 mg	1	10–22		
Church & Johnson, 1979	flurazepam	30 mg	10	9		↓
Oswald, 1979	flurazepam	30 mg	21	~10–18.5		

[a] Note: ↓ = impaired performance; ↑ = improved performance.
[b] Total response speed.
[c] High dose only.
[d] No distinction between motor and decision time.
[e] Both visual and auditory.

Hypnotics on Psychomotor Performance

Tapping rate	Card sorting (motor)	Card sorting (decision)	Symbol copying	Digit–symbol substitution test	Tracking test	Divided attention (visual)	Digit span	Auditory attentiveness
0	0	0	0	↓12 hr				
0	0	0	↓	↓12 hr				
↓c	↓	0		↓				
↓c	↓	0		↓				
↓	↓	0c	↓	0				
					↓19 hr, ↑34 hr ↓16 hr ↓19 hr, ↑34 hr			
	↓13 hr	↓13 hrc						
	0	↓13 hr						
	↓16 hrd			↓10 hr, low dose ↓16 hr, high dose				
	↓10 hrd			0				
					↓7 daysf	0		
					↓7 daysf	0		
					0 14 daysf	0		
					0 14 daysf	0		
	↓7th dayc	0		0				
0	0	0		0		0		
					↓	0		
					↓	↓		
						↓		
				↓i			0	
								↓

f Fixed speed test.
g All groups improved relative to predrug or preplacebo values.
h Decrease in one component (movement speed).
i Tolerance developed to this effect over 10 days.

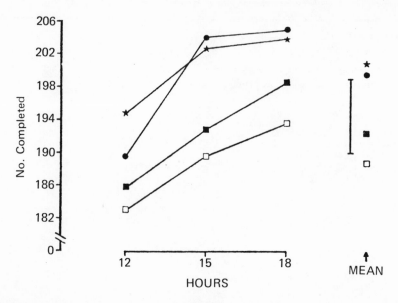

FIGURE 27. Mean scores on the symbol-copying test 12, 15, and 18 hr after placebo (star), 150 mg butabarbital (circle), 15 mg flurazepam (open square), and 30 mg flurazepam (closed square). (From Bond & Lader, 1973, by permission.)

1974), possibly a sign of loss of self-control. Similarly, pentobarbital (200 mg) can lead to initial deficits in adaptive tracking; and later, at 34 hr, there may actually be improved performance (Borland & Nicholson, 1975). Once again, however, this is a very selective kind of improvment—at this same time point, performance on reaction time test remained impaired. It has been suggested, incidentally, that improvements in performance following anxiolytics or hypnotics are more likely in untrained subjects, in whom anxiety may be inhibiting the learning process. Thus, more meaningful data may be obtained from well-trained subjects (Linnoila, 1978).

Another trend in the psychomotor data was that benzodiazepines tended to affect motor performance more, while barbiturates may also have more effects on measures of cognition (Bond & Lader, 1973; Joyce, Malpas, Rowan, & Scott, 1969; Malpas et al., 1970; Tansella, Siciliani, Burti, Schiavon, & Zimmermann-Tansella, 1975). Thus Malpas et al. (1975) found that the motor aspects of card dealing were impaired by nitrazepam, while this was unaffected by amobarbital, whereas both agents increased the decision time of card sorting. (Motor time was defined as the time necessary to sort a pile of identical cards into several stacks; decision time was the time necessary to sort different types of cards into several categories, minus the motor time.) Similarly, Bond and Lader

(1973) found that flurazepam affected the symbol-copying test (which is thought to reflect the motor aspects of the digit–symbol substitution test, or DSST), whereas butabarbital did not (Figure 27). Both drugs affected the full digit–symbol substitution test (Figure 28). The authors concluded, "whereas flurazepam may be exerting a motor impairment affecting both tasks or an initial coding impairment which wears off leaving a more prolonged motor impairment, butobarbitone mainly impairs the cognitive elements of the DSST . . ." (p. 234). Tansella *et al.* (1974) found that in anxious inpatients 1 week's treatment of 20 mg N-desmethyldiazepam produced a greater decrement in card sorting than either 200 mg amobarbital or placebo, although neither drug affected the digit–symbol substitution test. A similar study by the same group (Tansella *et al.*, 1975) suggested that although both drugs influenced other motor tests, amobarbital also decreased two-card decision time, a cognitive task. The two groups of drugs may thus have predilections for somewhat different types of deficits at clinical doses.

Drug-induced motor changes may be studied further by the use of an actograph, which measures the amount of spontaneous body movements. Crowley and Hydinger-Macdonald (1979) found that 30 mg flurazepam resulted in a 15.1% reduction in motor activity over the

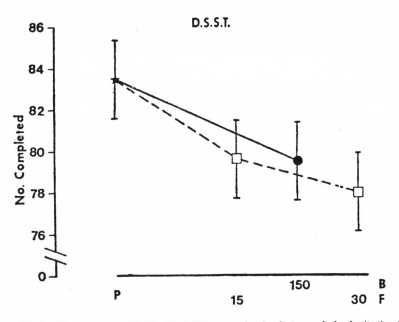

FIGURE 28. Mean scores and 0.05 critical differences for the digit–symbol substitution test 12 hr after drugs listed in Figure 27. (From Bond & Lader, 1973, by permission.)

following 24 hr in normal volunteers. A Profile of Mood States given during this same period was not affected by flurazepam. A comparable actograph study with a barbiturate is not available.

Two types of skills of particular concern are coordination and divided attention, because of tentative data suggesting that these skills may be predictive of the rate of driving accidents (Hakkinen, 1976). Effects on coordination, as reflected in adaptive tracking, are summarized in Table VIII. Saario and Linnoila (1976) compared daytime performance effects of 100 mg amobarbital and 30 mg flurazepam given at bedtime for 7–14 nights. It was found that after 7 nights both agents produced deficits in adaptive tracking, and the greatest effect was due to flurazepam (in fact, it impaired this test more than a drink of 0.5 g/kg ethanol given shortly before the morning testing). Neither Mandrax® nor glutethimide had significant effects on adaptive tracking. None of the drugs tested affected divided attention. In a similar paradigm, 10 mg nitrazepam for 1 week produced a small deficit in adaptive tracking, but clearly inhibited divided attention (Saario, Linnoila, & Maki, 1975). Diazepam 5 mg t.i.d. for 2 weeks was found to produce deficits in adaptive tracking but not divided attention (Linnoila, Saario, & Maki, 1974). If these skills are in fact predictive of driving safety, these results seem to raise the possibility of increased harm to persons taking hypnotics—particularly benzodiazepines.

It might be argued that although hypnotics produce a variety of performance deficits, these are offset by the improved functioning which follows a good night's sleep. Although this seems a reasonable possibility, there is at least some evidence against it. Bond and Lader (1972), in a study of normal subjects taking nitrazepam or butabarbital, found that the subject's estimate of the quality of a night's sleep was not related to his performance the next day. When either drug was given, however, the subjects felt that they had slept better, but their performance became worse. Similarly, in a study of patients with anxiety neurosis and insomnia, a week of treatment with 20 mg N-desmethyldiazepam produced better subjective sleep than did 200 mg amobarbital, but the patients on the former drug also had substantially poorer performance on two motor tasks. Bixler, Kales, Tan, and Kales (1973), in a study of two insomniacs, similarly reported that although total waking time was decreased by 100 mg secobarbital and 15 mg flurazepam, decision making in a card-sorting task was impaired. Saario and Linnoila (1976) found that 30 mg flurazepam given for 7 nights was experienced by the volunteers as inducing a "deep sleep," yet resulted in decreased performance on a tracking test. In contrast, a group of acutely sleep-deprived subjects felt that they were doing poorly, yet actually had no decreased performance.*

SUBJECTIVE EVALUATION OF DAYTIME PERFORMANCE

A review of the subjective evaluation of performance indicates that there is often little relationship to the actual objective findings. There is little evidence to suggest that this was specifically a greater problem with a particular class of drug. In some cases, patients correctly reported that performance was impaired after flurazepam or amobarbital (Saario & Linnoila, 1976). In others, subjects were unaware of their decreased performance with desmethyldiazepam (Tansella et al., 1975), or were aware of a deficit only with the higher dose of flunitrazepam, when in fact there were deficits with the lower dose also (Bond & Lader, 1975). Subjects throught that Mandrax® improved coordination and that glutethimide impaired it, when actually neither drug had significant effects (Saario & Linnoila, 1976). In a study in which diazepam (5 mg) was taken three times a day for 2 weeks, subjects thought their performance was impaired when in fact some tests (reaction time) had improved, while there were decrements in others (free-speed coordination test). In a carefully analyzed study, Borland and Nicholson (1975) demonstrated that subjects receiving pentobarbital (200 mg) or nitrazepam (10 mg) believed mistakenly that their performance on an adaptive tracking test had returned to normal by 16 hr (they also thought that performance after 30 mg flurazepam returned to normal at 16 hr, which it did between 16–19 hr). The authors established significant regression equations between actual performance on adaptive tracking tests and subjective assessment for pentobarbital and flurazepam, and for the latter drug the slope passed through the origin. A significant regression equation for nitrazepam could not be established. In other words, subjects receiving flurazepam could recognize the relative decrements in their performance and also relate it to the control level; subjects taking pentobarbital could identify relative changes in performance but could not relate it to their performance in the control period; subjects receiving nitrazepam could not even sense a relative change in performance.

Closely related but somewhat different from the subjective assessment of performance is the experiencing of side effects such as daytime sleepiness. Bond and Lader (1972), in comparing nitrazepam, and butabarbital, found that although high doses of both impaired perform-

*These subjects were kept awake until 3:00 A.M., then awakened hourly on the night before testing.

ance about equally 12 hr after administration, only the barbiturate produced a sensation of sleepiness at that time. Rather than considering this a drawback, however, they suggested that the sleepiness might serve as a useful warning of impaired abilities.

HYPNOTICS AND DRIVING

It is reasonable to wonder whether hypnotic-induced psychomotor deficits detected in the laboratory are translated into actual risk of harm. Perhaps the closest available source of data is studies on the relation of use of anxiolytics to traffic accidents. (These do, however, have to be considered with caution because of the potential role of anxiety or significant psychiatric disorder in the accident rates reported for drug users.) Ertama, Honkanen, and Kuosmanen (1978) found that pedestrians receiving psychotropic drugs in Helsinki were four to nine times more likely to be injured than sober controls. Murray (1960) reported that patients taking chlordiazepoxide had a tenfold increase in traffic accidents. Linnoila (1978) reported that among Finnish injured drivers, 5% were found to have diazepam in blood samples compared to 2% of controls. There is, then, some evidence that the use of benzodiazepines is associated with traffic injuries, but it should be emphasized that this may be numerically much smaller—perhaps one-fifth—than the problem of drinking and driving. There is also some reason to believe that anxiolytics and hypnotics in combination with ethanol may play a role in traffic accidents. Finkle (1969) reported that in one-quarter of 10,000 drinking driver investigations in Santa Clara County, California, there was evidence of concurrent use of a drug, of which 26% were anxiolytics or hypnotics. When drug determinations were performed on a subgroup—drivers who appeared intoxicated yet had blood ethanol concentrations usually too low to produce intoxication—about one-fifth were found to have significant concentrations of a drug, usually a barbiturate or glutethimide. In virtually all cases in which a drug was detected, ethanol was also present. In a Norwegian study of victims of nonfatal traffic accidents, 46% had blood ethanol concentrations suggestive of intoxication, 11% had significant concentrations of diazepam, and another 7% had both (Bo, Haffner, Langard, Trumpy, Bredesen, & Lunde, 1976). In contrast, only 3% of control subjects had blood levels of either substance, and no subject had both. Haffner, Bo, and Lunde (1974), in a study of 74 injured drivers in Norway, found that 9.4% had taken diazepam alone, and 10.8% had taken both diazepam and ethanol. In contrast, only 2% of control drivers had taken diazepam. Data such as these are clearly not conclusive, but do suggest that the interaction of anxiolytics and hypnotics may complicate the more common problem of drinking and driving. The toxic effects of this interaction are the subject of the next chapter.

SUMMARY AND CONCLUSIONS

It is clear that virtually all hypnotics continue to exert physiologic effects on the day(s) following their bedtime administration; this is hardly surprising insofar as the blood half-lives of most of these agents are substantially longer than 8 hr. This is reflected in altered patterns in the waking EEG as determined by frequency analysis studies, as well as in studies of psychomotor testing. Changes in the waking EEG often last longer than drug-induced alterations in performance. In some cases performance deficits are not seen after one dose, but appear after a week of treatment. Changes in performance are not always negative, and in fact, in some cases performance on specific tests has improved. (This may be related to anxiolytic effects which allow an untrained subject to learn a motor skill more easily.) Some authors have suggested that benzodiazepines produce relatively greater deficits in motor skills while barbiturates affect cognitive processes to a greater degree. Such conclusions are probably premature, however, as the testing procedures available are less specific than might be desired and the amount of data is not adequate. At this time it is probably more prudent to view the EEG and psychomotor test results as markers of the time course of central nervous system activity of these drugs, rather than to draw conclusions regarding the specific functions affected. There is also some question as to the practical significance of the performance deficits documented here. Some indirect evidence is derived from studies suggesting that use of benzodiazepine anxiolytics is associated with increased personal injury to drivers and pedestrians.

The subject's insight into his impaired performance is very unreliable; sometimes it is exaggerated and often is underestimated. The latter is, of course, a much greater problem insofar as a person unaware of his reduced capabilities might be more likely to come to harm. If side effects such as daytime sleepiness warn a person that he is still under the influence of a drug, perhaps they should not be considered an entirely negative experience.

Finally, it has sometimes been argued that the possibility of daytime performance deficits induced by hypnotics must be weighed against the benefits which come from improved sleep. It should be pointed out that it is not yet clear if the very real suffering of insomniacs is actually translated into objectively measured performance deficits; nor has there been any good demonstration that improving subjective sleep will aid performance. The small (insufficient) amount of data available suggests that many hypnotics improve the sensation of sleeping well, yet impair daytime functioning. (In contrast, one night's sleep deprivation had no effect on performance in one study.) The degree to which such deficits in psychomotor testing represent a real risk of harm from traffic accidents and similar situations needs to be carefully evaluated.

Interactions with Ethanol

Ethanol is often combined with hypnotics in an effort to improve sleep. Guilleminault, Spiegel, and Dement (1977), for instance, found that among 549 insomniacs in the Los Angeles area, 21% took ethanol plus a hypnotic "frequently." The two are also inadvertently combined whenever a person who has residual blood concentrations of a hypnotic from nightly use takes a drink during the day. This raises the possibility that their interaction may carry an increased risk either of toxicity or of injuries due to impaired coordination or judgment, for instance when driving (see Chapter 6). Ethanol is often taken in combination with hypnotics and other drugs in suicide attempts. (A combination of ethanol and a drug represents the second most common emergency room problem in the DAWN* program.) There is some reason to believe that concurrent ethanol use is often overlooked in patients who appear to be suffering from a drug toxicity. In one study, a pathology service looked for ethanol in blood samples which had been sent by physicians only for drug determinations (due to suspected toxic drug reactions). It was found that 19% of such samples were positive for ethanol as well (Hirsch, Valentour, Adelson, & Sunshine, 1973). Thus an examination of toxicity of hypnotics would be incomplete unless it also examined the interaction of these agents with ethanol. It might be well, however, first to mention briefly some basic principles of drug interactions.

*The Drug Abuse Warning Network (DAWN) monitors the number of "mentions" of drugs in 600 emergency rooms and 100 medical examiner's offices. It should be noted that what is counted is the number of incidents in which a drug is involved, not the number of patients (several drugs may be mentioned on one occasion; one patient may come to the emergency room several times). There is also some reason to believe that drug problems of "street people" are underrepresented in DAWN statistics (J. R. Cooper, 1977).

GENERAL CONSIDERATIONS

In Chapter 1 we pointed out that the magnitude and time course of a drug's effects are influenced by its absorption, distribution, and metabolism, as well as the (possibly changing) sensitivity of the target organ's receptors. One pharmacologic agent may influence any of these processes with respect to a second agent. An acute dose of ethanol, for instance, may inhibit the metabolism of hexobarbital (Chung & Brown, 1976), or may alter the distribution of glutethimide in the brain (Hetland & Couri, 1974). Such interactions between drugs may be manifested in effects which are *potentiated* (the total may be greater than the sum of their individual actions), *additive* (merely equal to the sum of their individual actions), or *antagonistic* (one drug may actually reduce the effects of another). In evaluating such interactions, several considerations should be kept in mind. The type of interaction may vary depending on:

The Dose. In one study, for instance, low doses of benzodiazepines and ethanol show no additive effects on sedation while at high doses there may be positive interactions (Zbinden & Randall, 1967).

The Duration of Administration. Pretreatment with a single dose of diazepam, for instance, may not affect the impaired attention measures induced by ethanol, whereas following administration of diazepam for 2 weeks, these ethanol-induced decrements may actually be antagonized (Linnoila, Saario, & Mattila, 1974).

Which Measure Is Examined. Depending on which performance test is used, the same two drugs may be reported to show either potentiation or no interaction (Linnoila, Saario, & Maki, 1974).

Which Drug Is Used. On some measures one drug (e.g., chlordiazepoxide) may interact with ethanol while another agent in the same pharmacologic class (e.g., diazepam) will not (Dundee, Howard, & Isaac, 1971).

Thus these interactions are very complex. Although recognizing these caveats, there remain some generalizations about the interactions of hypnotics and ethanol which have a bearing on the medical and social issues which are the concern here.

BARBITURATES

Studies on the interaction of barbiturates and ethanol show a relatively consistent, often fatal enhancement of toxic effects. When taken together, blood concentrations as low as 0.5 mg per 100 ml of secobarbital and 100 mg per 100 ml of ethanol may prove fatal; in contrast, fatal levels of secobarbital taken alone range from 1.1–6.0 mg per 100 ml and those of ethanol are thought to be in the range of at least 400 mg per 100 ml (Gupta & Kofoed, 1966; Ritchie, 1975). In rats, there is a dose-related decrease in the LD_{50} of several barbiturates as progressively greater doses of ethanol are given; in lower doses, sleeping time is prolonged when inactive amounts of both agents are given together (Wiberg, Coldwell, & Trenholm, 1969). The fatal results of this interaction in humans have been well documented (e.g., Bogan & Smith, 1968; Jetter & McLean, 1943; LeBreton & Garat, 1965). Another difficulty clinically is "accidental suicide," in which a person becomes confused by the ingestion of one substance and then inadvertently takes an overdose of the other (Teare, 1966).

The physiology of the interaction of barbiturates and ethanol is less well understood. In rats, brain levels of barbital and phenobarbital are increased by ethanol (Coldwell, Wiberg, & Trenholm, 1970). There are a variety of metabolic interactions between the two agents that might lead to such effects; in rats, ethanol lowers blood pressure and concomitant renal clearance of barbiturates, and lowers temperature, respiration, and blood pO_2 levels (Wiberg, Coldwell, & Trenholm, 1970). In other animal studies, acute ethanol administration inhibits the metabolic enzyme hexobarbital hydroxylase and may slow the decline in hexobarbital blood concentrations (Chung & Brown, 1976). One effect of inhibition of metabolism may be an accumulation of the barbiturate in the liver (Haacke, Johnsen, & Kolenda, 1976). Due to this alteration in distribution of barbiturates, the latter authors suggest that an inhibition of metabolism of the drug can even result in a lowering of blood concentrations. There is also evidence that measures of physiological interaction can occur at times that blood concentrations are not increased, suggesting some other process than merely retarding metabolism (Coldwell et al., 1970).

In chronic usage, in contrast to the acute interactions described above, cross-tolerance develops. Anaesthesiologists, for instance, often find that unusually large doses of barbiturates are necessary to induce sleep in alcoholics (Soehring & Schuppel, 1970). Similarly, barbiturate addicts are reported to have only slight intoxication following relatively large doses of ethanol (H.F. Fraser, Wikler, Isbell, & Johnson, 1957). The physiological basis of this cross-tolerance is not clear. As discussed in Chapter 3, one aspect of this may be the induction of hepatic microsomal drug-metabolizing enzymes, which then leads to more rapid metabolism of other drugs. Daily administration of phenobarbital or hexobarbital, for instance, has been reported to produce more rapid disappearance of ethanol from the blood (Fischer & Oelssner, 1960, 1961). In other studies, however, pretreatment with phenobarbital has been shown to increase total activity of ethanol-oxidizing enzymes, yet not affect ethanol clearance (Mezey, 1971). Chronic pretreatment with an inhibitor and two stimulators of hepatic enzymes (including phenobarbital) had little effect on ethanol clearance and metabolism, and no change in ethanol sleep time (Khanna & Kalant, 1970). In sum, the effect of barbiturates on ethanol blood clearance has varied in different studies. The rate of clearance has not always correlated well with the degree of induction of liver enzymes, and induction of enzymes has not always correlated with physiological effects. This leaves open the possibility of other interactions, such as one agent changing central nervous system sensitivity to the other (Khanna & Kalant, 1970).

When there is severe liver damage due to alcoholism, another problem appears—the alcoholic then becomes more sensitive to toxicity to barbiturates. This is of particular concern because of the alcoholic's propensity also to abuse barbiturates (Devenyi & Wilson, 1971).

In addition to alcoholics, others who may be particularly at risk of harm from the interaction of ethanol and barbiturates are patients with acute intermittent porphyria. Either agent alone can cause exacerbations of this illness (Fillipini, 1968; Harvey, 1975) by inducing increased amounts of the enzyme ALA synthetase (see Chapter 3). Studies in the rat suggest that these agents increase the amount of ALA synthetase in a manner greater than that which would be induced by merely additive effects (Held, 1977). An implication might be that the interaction of these two agents greatly increases the hazard of exacerbation for patients with acute intermittent porphyria.

BENZODIAZEPINES

Studies on the relation of benzodiazepines and ethanol have shown the widest range of results—from antagonism of sedative effects under some conditions to marked potentiation of psychomotor deficits in others. Many studies suggest that when low doses of benzodiazepines are taken in combination with a moderate amount of ethanol, there is little interaction. Lawton and Cahn (1963), for instance, found that diazepam 5 mg t.i.d. inhibited scores on several performance tests, but that there was little or no further deterioration after taking 3 ounces of 100-proof vodka. Similarly, there was no interaction on such tests as digit–symbol substitution, nor on physiological measures such as blood pressure and pulse with low doses of chlordiazepoxide and ethanol (Miller, D'Agostino, & Minsky, 1963).

In a few cases, the benzodiazepines have been reported to inhibit some effects of ethanol. Pretreatment of surgical patients with small doses of chlordiazepoxide, for instance, made it more difficult later to induce sleep with intravenous ethanol (Dundee *et al.*, 1971); this, however, is probably not generalizable to benzodiazepines as a whole, as this effect did not occur with diazepam. Similarly, the tranquilizing effect of chlordiazepoxide on rats (as measured by a conditioned avoidance behavior technique) may be negated by ethanol (Hughes, Rountree, & Forney, 1963).

In contrast to the previous studies, however, there is clear evidence that in many situations ethanol and benzodiazepines may have detrimental interactions (Linnoila & Mattila, 1973b; Molander & Duvhok, 1976; Morland, Setekleiv, Haffner, Stromsaether, Danielsen, & Holst Wethe, 1974). One study, for instance, found that ethanol (0.5 ml/kg) by itself had little effect on such measures as critical flicker fusion frequency and coordination, but markedly increased the detrimental effect of 10 mg or more of diazepam (Molander & Duvhok, 1976). (In a theme which may be becoming familiar, this was dose related and could not be generalized to other benzodiazepines: these effects were absent after 5 mg of diazepam, and ethanol did not enhance the effect of oxazepam on coordination.) In a study of skill with a driving stimulator, either 0.5 g/kg ethanol or a single dose of 10 mg diazepam caused an increase in collisions and ignoring of traffic rules during the next 2.5 hr. The combination of both agents increased these difficulties and also introduced a new type of problem— serious steering errors (Linnoila & Mattila, 1973a). Electrophysiological studies have also shown positive interactions between benzodiazepines and ethanol. EEG effects of 30 mg flurazepam may be substantially prolonged when taken in combination 0.8 g/kg of ethanol (Mendelson, Goodwin, Hill, & Reichman, 1976), although the clinical significance of such changes is unclear.

Perhaps because of the relatively long half-life of many benzodiazepines, it has become clear that taking ethanol during the daytime may potentiate effects of these agents even when they were last taken at bedtime; this may even present a bigger problem than with hypnotic barbiturates. Saario and Linnoila (1976), for instance, gave several hypnotics including 30 mg flurazepam and 100 mg amobarbital to normal volunteers for 14 nights, and performed daytime psychomotor tests at 7 and 14 days with and without giving 0.5 k/kg ethanol at 8:00 A.M. As was discussed in Chapter 6, both drugs impaired performance on a coordination test which involved using a steering wheel to keep a marker on a moving track. Flurazepam alone at night actually impaired coordination more than amobarbital alone, or even more than a placebo at night followed by ethanol in the morning. Perhaps most germane to the present discussion, ethanol given in the morning enhanced the deficit in patients receiving nighttime flurazepam, and did so to a lesser degree in patients

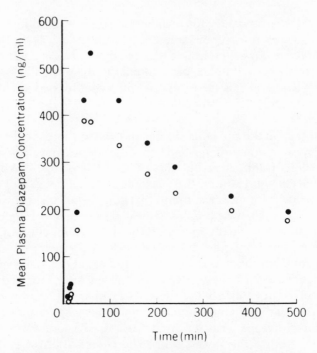

FIGURE 29. Mean plasma diazepam concentrations following ingestion of diazepam alone (open circles) and diazepam following pretreatment with ethanol 0.5 g/kg (closed circles) in eight normal volunteers. (From McLeod *et al.*, 1977, by permission.)

receiving amobarbital. In a similar paradigm, 10 mg nitrazepam had no effects on daytime coordination, but enhanced the decrement due to daytime ethanol (Saario *et al.*, 1975).

Overdoses of large quantities of benzodiazepines are generally relatively benign, and deaths from these agents when taken alone have rarely if ever been confirmed (Chapter 5). There have been rare reports of deaths consequent to overdoses of a combination of chlordiazepoxide (Rada *et al.*, 1975) or nitrazepam (Torry, 1976) plus ethanol, suggesting perhaps some toxic interaction at high doses.

The physiologic basis of the interactions of benzodiazepines and ethanol is not clear. There is some evidence that coadministration raises blood chlordiazepoxide concentrations (Linnoila, Otterstrom, & Anttila, 1974). Data on the possibility of altered absorption of diazepam has been contradictory (Linnoila & Mattila, 1974; Linnoila, Otterstrom, & Anttila, 1974; McLeod, Giles, Patzalek, Thiessen, & Sellers, 1977). Absorption of diazepam appears to be affected differently by various alcoholic beverages (Linnoila, 1978), and is enhanced when diazepam is administered as a powder (Hayes, Pablo, Radomski, & Palmer, 1977). McLeod *et al.* (1977) reported that coadministration of diazepam tablets and ethanol enhances diazepam concentrations, but attributed this to a decreased initial volume of distribution (Figures 29 and 30). Linnoila, Otterstrom, and Anttila (1974) reported no change in diazepam concentrations. They suggested that if in fact there is a behavioral interaction but no increase in diazepam blood concentrations, the site of interaction might be at receptors in the central nervous system. Altered distribution of diazepam must also be considered; pretreatment with ethanol may substantially increase brain concentrations of diazepam in the rat (Whitehouse, Paul, Coldwell, & Thomas, 1975).

In summary, studies of the interactions of benzodiazepines and ethanol have had varied results. In low doses, some studies have reported no decrement in performance and in some special circumstances the agents may even be antagonistic. Ascione (1978), in summarizing this area, suggests that diazepam seems to have the most positive interactions with ethanol, while chlordiazepoxide and oxazepam have the least. In the majority of studies, however, increased decrements in performance have been produced when these agents are taken together, and in large doses deaths have occurred.

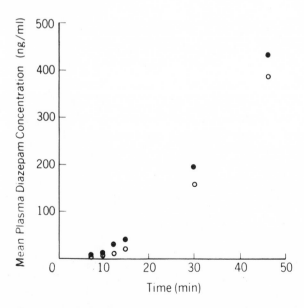

FIGURE 30. Mean plasma diazepam concentrations in the first 45 min following ingestion of diazepam alone (open circles) and diazepam following pretreatment with ethanol 0.5 g/kg (closed circles) in eight normal volunteers. (From McLeod *et al.*, 1977, by permission.)

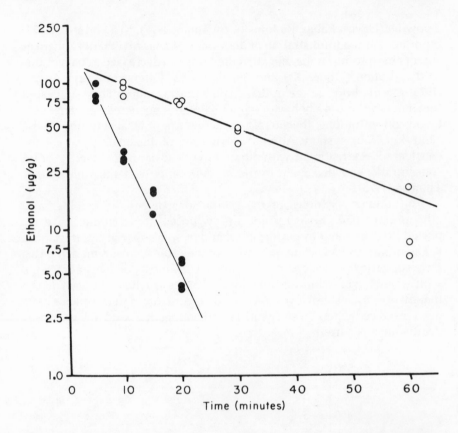

FIGURE 31. Concentrations of ethanol at various times after intraperitoneal administration of 139 mg/kg ethanol (closed circles) and an equimolar mixture of 139 mg/kg ethanol and 452 mg/kg trichloroethanol (open circles) in mice. A decrease in rate of disappearance of ethanol also occurs when it is coadministered with the parent compound, chloral hydrate. (From Gessner, 1973, by permission.)

NONBARBITURATE, NONBENZODIAZEPINE HYPNOTICS

Chloral Hydrate

Chlorate hydrate and ethanol have potentiating effects on sleep time in mice (Gessner & Cabana, 1964). In humans this combination has been referred to as "knockout drops" or the "Micky Finn" (Sharpless, 1965), which have been taken with fatal results (Shah, Clancy, & Iber, 1972). The potentiating effects of this combination are the basis of advocacy for the use of chloral alcoholate, a hypnotic which is rapidly metabolized in the body into chloral hydrate and ethanol, and whose effects are indistinguishable from an equivalent mixture of these two agents (Gessner & Cabana, 1967).

The metabolic pathways of chloral hydrate and ethanol are closely intertwined. As discussed in Chapter 3, chloral hydrate is rapidly reduced to trichloroethanol, which is thought to have the major central nervous system depressant effects (E.K. Marshall & Owens, 1954). This reaction, and the oxidation of ethanol to acetaldehyde, are mediated by alcohol dehydrogenase. Trichloroethanol itself has been reported to cause inhibition of ethanol oxidation (Friedman & Cooper, 1960). Gessner (1973) has demonstrated that coadministration results in a decrease in ethanol disappearance (Figure 31), and an increase in the rate of conversion of chloral hydrate to trichloroethanol, and believed that the latter phenomenon is primarily responsible for the potentiating effects (see also Freeman & Schulman, 1970).

Methaqualone

The concomitant use of methaqualone[*] and ethanol is of particular interest in that in some drug-taking subcultures it is believed that this produces a particularly pleasant sensation. Unfortunately, it is also particularly dangerous ("Mixing Mandrax and Alcohol," 1973; Norheim, 1974). In one study of methaqualone poisoning, 23% of the patients had also consumed ethanol (Ruedy, 1973). Similarly, Ostrenga (1973) found that most methaqualone deaths occurred when the drug was taken in combination with ethanol. Although results have varied somewhat, many studies in humans do suggest increased toxicity (Gerald & Schwirian, 1973; Inaba et al., 1973). Four hours after coadministration to rats, concentrations of methaqualone in blood, kidney, fat, and brain are higher than in controls, possibly due to reduced biliary excretion of methaqualone (Whitehouse, Peterson, Paul, & Thomas, 1977).

Glutethimide

Enhanced toxicity with combinations of glutethimide and ethanol are well documented. In rats, a single oral dose of 250 mg/kg glutethimide produces no deaths, but when combined with 3 g/kg of ethanol results in

---

[*]This is also often taken as Mandrax®, a fixed combination with the antihistamine diphenhydramine hydrochloride.

a 40% mortality (Hetland & Couri, 1974). In dogs, central depressant effects and toxicity are enhanced by combining the two agents, and blood concentrations of each are increased 12 hr later (Melville, Joran, & Douglas, 1966). Blood and whole brain concentrations of gluthethimide are enhanced in rats by simultaneous administration of ethanol (Figure 32). Following oral administration of glutethimide and intraperitoneal ethanol, the regional distribution of brain glutethimide changes, favoring an increase in the pons–medulla and cerebellum (Hetland & Couri, 1974). (This may be related to the observations of ataxia and fatal respiratory depression seen clinically.) In normal humans the simultaneous ingestion of both agents results in enhancement of blood ethanol concentrations and a slight decrease in plasma glutethimide (Mould, Curry, & Binns, 1972). (The possibility would seem to exist that the later phenomenon is related to increased concentrations in various other tissues.) In a manner analogous to that of the benzodiazepines, results of various

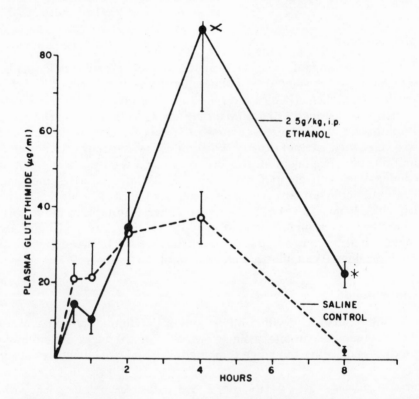

FIGURE 32. The effect of ethanol (2.5 g/kg i.p.) on plasma concentrations of glutethimide (500 mg/kg orally) in rats. (From Hetland & Couri, 1974, by permission.)

performance tests vary with the individual test. In tracking and finger-tapping tests, the greatest impairment was after glutethimide alone, and this was reversed by simultaneous administration of ethanol. On the other hand, a reaction time test was insensitive to ethanol or glutethimide alone, but was markedly impaired by a combination of both agents (Mould *et al.*, 1972). In the Saario and Linnoila (1976) study described previously, nighttime administration of glutethimide or Mandrax® did not enhance daytime coordination deficits induced by ethanol.

SUMMARY AND CONCLUSIONS

Because hypnotics and ethanol are often combined both in usual practice and in overdose, it behooves us to be aware of the consequences of their interaction. The results of studies in this area are profoundly affected by dose, duration of treatment, the particular measure used, and other variables, so generalizations are very risky. The enhancement of toxicity from the acute ingestion of barbiturates and ethanol is well recognized. In chronic usage, cross-tolerance develops (although alcoholics with severe liver damage may have increased sensitivity to barbiturates). Among the benzodiazepines, diazepam seems to interact with ethanol substantially in terms of performance deficits, while chlordiazepoxide and oxazepam do so to a lesser degree. There is some evidence that with repeated nocturnal use, flurazepam and nitrazepam enhance coordination deficits when ethanol is consumed the next morning. Nocturnal Mandrax® and glutethimide have been reported not to affect such daytime ethanol-induced deficits in one study. These agents and chloral hydrate do, however, greatly enhance clinical toxicity when large doses are taken in combination with ethanol.

Hypnotic Dependence

It is well to consider the risk of inducing dependence whenever a patient is started on hypnotics. Dependence, as used in this chapter, refers to an interaction of a person, a drug, and the environment resulting in habitual consumption (World Health Organization, 1969, 1975).* Qualities which are often related include tolerance and physical dependence. *Tolerance* refers to a diminished response to a given quantity of drug on repeated use, which may lead to increasing the dosage progressively to maintain the desired effect. *Physical dependence* refers to the production of a characteristic group of symptoms when the administration of a drug is discontinued. (Upon withdrawal of high chronic doses of barbiturates, for instance, there can occur a symptom complex including seizures, fever, and delirium.) The relationship of tolerance and physical dependence to the compulsion habitually to consume a drug is not clear. A World Health Organization (1975) Scientific Group has emphasized that neither quality is essential to dependence, pointing out that such drugs as nalorphine and cyclazocine may produce both tolerance and physical dependence but do not induce drug-seeking behavior in animals or man. Conversely, cocaine and some stimulants do not produce physical dependence, yet may produce a strong craving.

---

*World Health Organization (1969) definition: "Drug Dependence: A state, psychic and sometimes also physical, resulting from the interaction between a living organism and a drug, characterized by behavioral and other responses that always include a compulsion to take the drug on a continuous or periodic basis in order to experience its psychic effects, and sometimes to avoid the discomfort of its absence. Tolerance may or may not be present. A person may be dependent on more than one drug" (p. 6).

CLASSICAL DRUG ABUSE

The aspect of hypnotic dependence which has received most attention has been the more obvious forms of drug abuse in which individuals habitually take hypnotics for essentially nonmedical reasons, such as the induction of euphoria or some other gratifying state. Often accompanying this is a lifestyle dominated by concern with obtaining and taking drugs. Historically, the introduction of virtually every hypnotic has been followed within a few years by reports of abuse. Barbital, the first clinically used barbiturate, for instance, was introduced in 1903 and the first description of abuse was in 1904 (Table IX). It has been estimated that there are 200,000–2,000,000 abusers of sedative–hypnotics in the United States (W.R. Martin, 1977). In 1976, there were 10,764 admissions for barbiturate abuse at federally funded drug treatment centers, and there were another 6442 for other sedative–hypnotics or anxiolytics (Cooper, 1977). (In order to keep a sense of perspective, it should be noted that there were 219,064 admissions for all other drugs.) Particularly worri-

TABLE IX

Year of Clinical Introduction of Sedative and Hypnotic Drugs, and
First Abuse Reports[a]

Generic name	Year of clinical introduction	First abuse report
Bromide	1838	Seguin, 1877
Chloral hydrate	1869	Kelp, 1875
Paraldehyde	1882	Krafft-Ebing, 1887
Barbiturate	1903	Fernandez & Clarke, 1904
Ethinamate	1954	Brouschek & Feuerlein, 1956
Ethchlorvynol	1955	Cahn, 1959
Glutethimide	1955	Battegay, 1957
Meprobamate	1955	Lemere, 1956
Methaqualone	1955	Ewart & Priest, 1967
Methyprylon	1955	Jensen, 1960
Clomethiazole	1959	Tengblad, 1961
Chlordiazepoxide	1960	Guile, 1963
Diazepam	1962	Czerwenka-Wenkstetten, Hofman, & Krypsin-Exnec, 1965
Nitrazepam	1965	Johnson & Clift, 1968
Oxazepam	1965	Selig, 1966
Flurazepam	1970	Swanson et al., 1973
Lorazepam	1975	Korsgaard, 1976
Clorazepate	1972	Allgulander & Borg, in press

[a] From Allgulander (1978), by permission.

some is the possible association of barbiturate abuse with crime. Ecker-man, Bates, Bachel, and Poole (1971) reported that 16% of individuals arrested in several cities were currently using barbiturates. Tinklenberg, Murphy, Murphy, Daryl, Roth, and Kopell (1974), in a study of adolescent offenders, found that secobarbital and ethanol abuse were related to assaultive behavior. Public attention to this very real social and medical problem resulting from the use of hypnotics is of course vital, but there has been a tendency to focus here, perhaps to the neglect of other, less dramatic areas of concern. Among these is the development of dependence which is clearly *within* the context of medical practice.

DEPENDENCE IN MEDICAL PRACTICE

Two sorts of clinical pictures are of concern here. In the first, the patient seeking relief from insomnia takes progressively larger amounts of medication; this may lead to a self-perpetuating state in which he continues to experience disturbed sleep while taking substantially more than the recommended doses. The second includes patients taking recommended dosages regularly for prolonged periods.

Dependence on Extremely Large Doses

In clinical lore the first type of patient goes to a physician for insomnia and initially experiences relief with a hypnotic. He finds that the effectiveness quickly dissipates and responds by increasing the dosage, sometimes with and sometimes without the consent of the physician. Often the patient will add ethanol to the regimen. He may report having had unsuccessful attempts to discontinue all his medicines all at once. (For descriptions of this condition see Dement *et al.*, 1975a; Hauri, 1977; A. Kales, Bixler, Tan, Scharf, & Kales, 1974.) Hypnotic abuse in this manner has been noted to occur somewhat more often in women, particularly of middle age (Allgulander, 1978; Swanson, Weddige, & Morse, 1973; Wissler, 1969). In a study of 55 patients hospitalized for hypnotic dependence in Stockholm, 44 indicated that they had initially started on these drugs because of insomnia (Allgulander, 1978). Most commonly they obtained their large quantities of medication by seeking parallel prescriptions from two or more doctors (Allgulander, 1978; Swanson *et al.*, 1973; Whitlock, 1970).

It is not known how often this desperate clinical picture appears, although the data of Clift (1975b) suggest it is relatively uncommon compared to the number of persons started on hypnotics. In sleep disorder clinics where, if anything, their numbers might be expected to be particularly large, they have been reported to comprise 4–6.5% of patients complaining of insomnia (Billiard *et al.*, 1978; Dement *et al.*, 1975b; Hauri, 1976). Among psychiatric inpatients in various cities the incidence of sedative–hypnotic abuse has been reported to be up to about 10% (Allgulander, 1978).

The sleep EEGs of patients chronically taking dosages substantially larger than the therapeutic range have been reported by A. Kales, Bixler, Tan, Scharf, and Kales (1974). In terms of sleep latency and total waking time their sleep is no better than that of chronic insomniacs who are not receiving medication, and REM sleep percentage may be lower (also see Kales, 1971).

When an attempt is made to withdraw the hypnotic, the patient who has been taking these very large doses will often experience severe sleep disturbance (A. Kales, Bixler, Tan, Scharf, & Kales, 1974; Oswald & Priest, 1965). (In quantities greater than 600 mg/day of a hypnotic barbiturate, a clinical withdrawal syndrome including seizures and delirium may appear.) The appropriate treatment as outlined by A. Kales, Bixler, Tan, Scharf, and Kales, (1974) is gradually to withdraw the hypnotic at a rate of one therapeutic dose every 5 or 6 days, while being very supportive.

Prolonged Use of Recommended Doses

Incidence and Contributing Factors

Of equal concern are patients who are dependent in the sense that they seek to take recommended doses for extended periods. As discussed in Chapter 2, perhaps 1–3% of the population is actually taking hypnotics nightly for at least several months. Very few data are available on how this has come to pass. Some of the most thoughtful work has been done by Clift (1975a,b), in reports from a group general practice in the area of Manchester, Great Britain. In one study he prospectively followed 50 patients with a primary complaint of insomnia, and who had not received hypnotics for at least 3 months. All were given a nonbarbiturate hypnotic, usually nitrazepam (Figure 33). It was found that 4 years later, 15–20% were still taking hypnotics regularly. In attempting to distinguish which factors might be predictive of dependence, he found that no specific indication for the use of hypnotics (in their classification, medical or surgical, psychiatric, or "onset insomnia") was more likely to be associated with dependence. The Cornell Medical Index, although indicating a great deal of psychological disturbance in all the subjects, did not distinguish those who later became dependent. A classification of per-

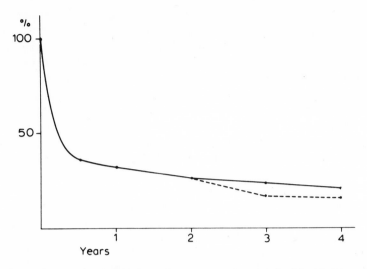

FIGURE 33. Proportion of patients continuing to receive a nonbarbiturate hypnotic after starting treatment in a prospective study. (From Clift, 1975a, by permission.)

sonality types indicated that the hysterical personality was associated with the development of dependence.

In a second study, Clift (1975c) prospectively compared the consequences of starting 102 patients on a single nightly tablet of either a barbiturate (100 mg amobarbital) or nonbarbiturate (5 mg nitrazepam). This time it was found that even though all patients were encouraged to discontinue hypnotics as soon as possible, 8% had taken them continuously at 2-year follow-up, and an additional 7% were taking them at follow-up but had been off medication sometime previously. Clift then assessed factors associated with the development of dependence, which he defined as continuous drug consumption 6 weeks after the initial prescription (this occurred in 49 patients). Approximately equal numbers were receiving amobarbital and nitrazepam after 6 weeks. During this time, no patients increased their medications beyond two tablets nightly; those who did increase their dose to two tablets were more likely to become dependent, however. Patients who had received a hypnotic (barbiturate or nonbarbiturate) in the past were more likely to become dependent. Males were most likely to be dependent when 33–44 years old, while for females it was associated with the 45- to 64-year-old group. Patients with mixed insomnias* were more likely to become dependent

*This group included several types of patients, predominantly those with multiple awakenings either alone or accompanied by difficulty falling asleep or early-morning awakenings.

than those who only had difficulty with falling asleep or early-morning awakenings. Dependence was significantly associated with the persistence of the original indications for the medication (these were classified as medical or psychiatric disorders, "normal psychological" insomnia related to anxiety-producing life events, or a relatively isolated complaint of difficulty falling asleep). On the other hand, almost half of the nondependent patients continued to have the original associated condition at 6-week follow-up. Thus the persistence of the original indication may contribute to prolonged hypnotic use, but it is clearly only one of many important variables. Although a history of overt treated psychiatric illness or abnormal personality were not associated with dependence, the nonpsychiatric patients who had high scores on a symptom-sign checklist (Personal Disturbance Scale of Foulds) were more likely to become dependent. Interestingly, 60% of the patients with "normal psychological" insomnia (related to overt anxiety about specific life events) were still taking hypnotics 6 weeks later.

An earlier study of Johnson and Clift (1968) indicates the contribution of hypnotic use during hospitalization to later chronic use. In a study of 97 patients who were receiving repeat hypnotic prescriptions for over 3 months (1.3% of their group practice), it was found that 21.6% had started their medication while hospitalized (in 12 of the 21 cases for a medical illness and in 9 cases for a psychiatric disorder). Pursuing this finding by following up patients in a Manchester hospital, they found that 5% of the psychiatric patients and 3% of the medical and surgical patients were receiving a hypnotic 18 months after discharge. In their own group of 97 patients, the most common indication for prescribing a hypnotic was insomnia related to a medical illness (48 cases), followed by psychiatric illness (30 cases), usually associated with abnormal personality traits. Only 2 patients of the 97 were found to increase dosage markedly with ultimate difficulties with intoxication.

Aside from the studies of Clift (1975a,b) there has been virtually no work on personality traits or psychopathology leading to prolonged hypnotic use, although there are a number of studies relating to more classic drug abuse (e.g., H.E. Hill, Haertzen, & Yamahiro, 1968; Rado, 1933; Wikler & Rasor, 1953). Authors such as Cocchi and Tornati (1977) have emphasized the role of depression, to which chronic drug taking may be a maladaptive response, in the development of dependence. Sometimes prolonged self-medication has been viewed as an attempt to replace a chronic (perhaps congenital) neurochemical deficiency (Cocchi & Tornati, 1977).

Other considerations must include the role of the physician who prescribes hypnotics for durations for which their efficacy is at least questionable. Relatively little is known about how education, attitudes, and other factors affect how physicians prescribe hypnotics, although some interesting work has come out on traits related to appropriateness of prescribing other classes of drugs (Stolley, Becker, Lasagna, McEvilla, & Sloane, 1972). Sociological factors such as acceptance of the use of medications in different socioeconomic groups may play a role in long-term drug use.

Drug Qualities Related to Prolonged Use

We have established, then, that a large percentage of hypnotics users go on to consume generally accepted therapeutic dosages for substantial periods, and we have commented on the clinical indications, personality of the patient, the role of hospitalization, and other factors associated with prolonged usage. Aspects of the drug effects which might lead to prolonged usage may be divided into two categories: (1) those not necessarily related to sleep; and (2) those related to their sleep-inducing properties.

Nonsleep Effects. These are largely beyond the scope of this work, but some comments are in order. It seems clear that there is some self-reinforcing quality about the administration of hypnotics. A classical paradigm in which this is demonstrated involves self-injection studies with monkeys and dogs, in which the animals voluntarily continue to inject themselves with barbiturates and nonbenzodiazepine, nonbarbiturate hypnotics to the point of unconsciousness (Fraser & Jasinsky, 1977). The benzodiazepines are likewise self-administered, although to a lesser degree (Table X). It has been commented that factors which favor "psychic dependence" include rapid onset of action, euphoriant effects, lack of unpleasant side effects, and the ability rapidly to induce a state of "total oblivion" (Zbinden & Randall, 1967), qualities shared by most hypnotics.

Sleep-Related Effects. Among the possibilities here are that patients continue to take hypnotics because: (1) the hypnotics provide relief of the sleep disturbance, a strong incentive to continue medication; (2) the hypnotics induce a sleep disturbance leading to continued hypnotic use; (3) the presence of a withdrawal syndrome leads to prolonged use. These hypotheses will now each be considered in turn. It will become apparent that there are insufficient data to confirm or refute any of these, and that they are by no means mutually exclusive. Nevertheless they are each supported by tantalizing but inadequate data and generally are testable.

POSSIBILITY 1: Hypnotics Provide Long-Term Benefits. We simply do

TABLE X

Summary of Dependence Liability Tests with Sedative/Hypnotic Agents in Rhesus Monkeys[a]

Drugs	Complete suppression doses in cross-physical dependence test[b] (mg/kg)	Physical dependence-producing test[b]	Self-administration test[b]	Overt signs of drug effect during self-administration
Pentobarbital-Na	25 (i.v.)	Positive	Markedly reinforcing (i.v., i.g.)[f]	Coma
Alcohol	4000 (p.o.)	Positive	Markedly reinforcing (i.g.)	Coma
Chloroform	Subanesthetic dose (inhal.)	Untested	Markedly reinforcing[c] (inhal.)	Coma
Meprobamate	200 (p.o.)	Positive	Untested	Untested
Diazepam	5 (p.o.)	Positive	Moderately reinforcing (i.v.)	Ataxia
Chlordiazepoxide	20 (p.o.)	Positive	Mildly reinforcing (i.v., i.g.)	Ataxia
Oxazolam	20 (p.o.)	Positive	Mildly reinforcing (i.g.)	Sedation
Benzoctamine	Not suppressed	Negative	Mildly reinforcing[d] (i.g.)	Sedation
Perlapine	Not suppressed	Negative	Not reinforcing (i.g.)	None
Chlorpromazine	Not suppressed	Negative	Not reinforcing[e] (i.v.)	None

[a] Abbreviations used: i.v., intravenous; p.o., oral; i.g., intragastric; inhal., inhalation. From Fraser and Jininsky (1977) by permission.
[b] For details, see text.
[c] Quoted from a previous study (Yanagita & Takahashi, 1970).
[d] Reinforcement observed in only 1 of 6 monkeys.
[e] Quoted from a previous study (Deneau et al., 1969).
[f] Route given in parentheses.

not know if this is the case. The systematic studies have generally been for 28 days or less, and even these have reported quantitatively modest improvements in various EEG or clinical measures. These studies are, of course, performed on *groups* of patients; the possibility exists that although hypnotic effectiveness quickly dissipates in most patients, certain individual subjects continue (for as yet unknown reasons) to obtain lasting benefits. It may also be that hypnotics are providing long-term benefits not adequately measured by the available studies (see discussion in Chapter 4). Population studies such as that by Balter and Bauer (1975) suggest that perhaps 80% of patients find that their hypnotic "helps" substantially. Similarly, Clift (1975c) found that only 6 of 102 patients on either amobarbital or nitrazepam felt that these hypnotics "had not improved sleep to their satisfaction."

PossibiLITY 2: Hypnotics Induce a Self-Perpetuating Sleep Disturbance. As discussed before, it seems clear that very large chronic dosages of many hypnotics do indeed perpetuate a sleep disturbance. It is not clear if this is the case in chronic use of therapeutic doses. Certainly there are persistent changes in the sleep EEG, for instance, decreased slow-wave sleep with nitrazepam (Adam *et al.*, 1976) or flurazepam (Dement *et al.*, 1978). However, it is not known if such changes can be translated into a sensation of poor sleep.

Another possibility is that some hypnotics disturb sleep each night by a "partial drug withdrawal" phenomenon, which occurs late at night when the drug concentrations have decreased due to metabolism or excretion (A. Kales, Malmstrom, Scharf, & Rubin, 1969). This effect was suggested by Mullin, Kleitman, and Cooperman (1933), who observed that after ethanol ingestion restlessness was decreased early at night, but increased after several hours. Similarly, Ogunremi *et al.* (1973) found that restlessness as defined by the EEG (shifts to Stage 1 or awake) followed this same pattern in the fifth week of administration of amobarbital to four normal volunteers. A biphasic effect on REM sleep, with an initial decrease followed by an increase late at night, has been reported with ethanol (Knowles, Laverty, & Kuechler, 1968; Williams & Salamy, 1972), barbiturates (A. Kales, Preston, Tan, & Allen, 1970), and nitrazepam (Adam *et al.*, 1976). Whether such a "partial drug withdrawal" effect is reflected in a subjective sensation of sleep disturbance is of course not known.

Most sleep researchers believe that in some cases patients can be successfully treated for their insomnia by weaning them off their hypnotics and being supportive during the initial period of drug withdrawal. In one case series of 75 patients complaining of insomnia from a variety of causes, Billiard *et al.* (1976) found that in four cases the insomnia cleared when hypnotics were withdrawn. There are not yet adequate data on what percentage of insomniacs without other associated disorders actually do benefit from this procedure.

Possibility 3: The Presence of a Withdrawal Syndrome Leads to Prolonged Drug Use. From the areas of classical drug abuse, there is evidence that the potential of severe withdrawal syndromes may be differentiated from the self-reinforcing qualities of a drug. Heroin addicts who have been off drugs for substantial periods of time may feel a strong craving (World Health Organization, 1975), and drugs such as cocaine which do not produce a withdrawal syndrome may nonetheless be very appealing to some individuals for repeated use (World Health Organization, 1975). As mentioned earlier, withdrawal from the very large doses of the classical drug abuser may result in severe withdrawal syndromes, which for barbiturates may begin with anxiety, tremors, and nausea, and later lead to seizures, delirium, hyperpyrexia, and death (Eddy, Halbach, Isbell, & Seever, 1966; A. Fraser & Jasinsky, 1977; see Table XI). Studies by H.F. Fraser, Wilker, Essig, and Isbell (1958), and Essig and Fraser (1958), suggest that at least 600 mg of pentobarbital or secobarbital daily for at least a month are necessary before such symptoms appear; daily doses of 400 mg for 3 months were not followed by these major symptoms. Extremely large doses of benzodiazepines such as 300 mg per day of chlordiazepoxide and up to 1200 mg per day of diazepam (Hollister, Bennett, Kimbell, Savage, & Overall, 1963; Hollister, Motzenbecher, & Degan, 1961) may also lead to severe withdrawal symptoms.

Although abrupt withdrawal from high doses of hypnotics (equivalent to 600 mg or less of a hypnotic barbiturate) will not produce the massive syndromes described above, they certainly produce disturbed sleep (A. Kales, Bixler, Tan, Scharf, & Kales, 1974; Oswald & Priest, 1966), and this is also thought to occur to some degree during withdrawal from therapeutic doses. As we will see, the role of this withdrawal sleep disturbance in the persistence of drug use is as problematic as the role of major withdrawal syndromes in traditional drug abuse. It is not entirely clear how often sleep disturbance occurs following therapeutic doses; it is certainly not invariable. Clift (1975c, and personal communication) found that of the 53 patients who successfully discontinued hypnotic medications, 13% experienced clinical disturbance of their sleep upon withdrawal; among his 49 dependent patients, 42% reported insomnia during attempted withdrawal. Although roughly the same number of patients ultimately became dependent on nitrazepam and amobarbital, insomnia during attempted withdrawal appeared in 64% of the former and only 25% of the latter. These figures seem to suggest that although withdrawal insomnia may contribute to hypnotic dependence, there is not a simple relationship, and other factors need to be considered.

TABLE XI

Summary of Data on Relationship of Dosage of Secobarbital or Pentobarbital to Intensity of Physical Dependence[a]

Patients			Daily dose of barbiturate (g)	Days of intoxication in hospital	Number of patients having symptoms		
Total number	Number receiving				Convulsions	Delirium	Minor symptoms of significant degree
	Seco-barbital	Pento-barbital					
18	16	2	0.9–2.2	32–144	14	12	18
5	5		0.8	42–57	1	0	5
18	18		0.6	35–57	2	0	9
18	10	8	0.4	90	0	0	1
2	1	1	0.2	365	0	0	0

[a] From Fraser & Jasinsky (1977), by permission.

In the past, much emphasis has been placed on the "rebound" increase in REM sleep that occurs during the withdrawal period, and the implication has often been drawn that it is in fact the increased REM which causes this feeling of disturbed sleep and nightmares. It is not clear if this is so. Although not well documented, the impression of some investigators who have deprived subjects of REM sleep by nonpharmacologic means (awakening them when they enter REM sleep) is that the recovery nights (when there is a REM rebound) are often subjectively felt to be restful.

Furthermore, at clinical doses of hypnotics, even the occurrence of the REM rebound is inconsistent: it may not occur, for instance, after 200 mg of phenobarbital for 5 nights or 200 mg of secobarbital for 8 nights (I. Feinberg, Hibi, Cavness, & March, 1974), 100 mg secobarbital for 2 weeks (A. Kales, Hauri, Bixler, & Silverfarb, 1976), 1 mg flunitrazepam or 10 mg nitrazepam for 1 week, or 0.5 mg triazolam for 2 weeks (A. Kales, Scharf, & Kales, 1978). During the period of withdrawal from these benzodiazepines, EEG measures of disturbed sleep (increased sleep latency and intermittent awakening) may occur in the absence of a REM rebound. In sum, the nonpharmacologic REM deprivation studies, and the observation of disturbed sleep without REM rebound upon cessation of some hypnotics, suggest that sleep disturbance after drug withdrawal is not simply due to enhanced REM sleep.

SUMMARY AND CONCLUSIONS

The studies described here indicate that when patients are started on hypnotics, a large percentage (possibly 15–20% in one series) may be taking the first steps toward long-term hypnotic use. In an unknown but probably small percentage, a tendency for a loss of effectiveness (and other factors) may lead patients to increase dosage to the point where they are consuming large quantities, yet continue to sleep poorly. The appropriate treatment here is gradual withdrawal, education, and emotional support.

A much more common situation is the patient who chronically takes hypnotics in doses not necessarily exceeding the therapeutic range. Studies of this phenomenon by Clift (1975a,b) suggest the following tentative conclusions: prolonged hypnotic use may often begin when it is prescribed during hospitalization for medical or psychiatric illness and is then continued after discharge. Dependence may also often result when hypnotics are given to an apparently stable person who seems to be having a reasonable degree of anxiety and insomnia in response to a perceived stress. It may be less likely that persons with an isolated complaint of difficulty falling asleep, without accompanying illness or stress, will become dependent. In terms of the specific complaint, a patient with difficulty only in falling asleep or awakening early may be less likely to become dependent than one with multiple awakenings or a mixture of symptoms. Patients who raise their dosage from one to two tablets per night early in treatment may be more likely to become dependent. Although a history of overt psychiatric illness or abnormal personality does not clearly increase the likelihood of later dependence, there is a tendency for dependence-prone patients to score higher on a test of personal disturbance. Patients in medical practice who are started on nitrazepam are as likely to become dependent as those receiving amobarbital.

The sources of prolonged hypnotic use in the context of medical practice are unclear, but probably they involve nonpharmacologic factors (e.g., personality of the patient, attitude of the physician), pharmacologic properties not necessarily related to sleep (e.g., euphoria), and aspects of the drug's hypnotic properties. Among the latter are the possibilities that hypnotics are providing adequate relief from insomnia, that hypnotics themselves induce a self-perpetuating sleep disturbance, or that the sleep disturbance upon withdrawal leads to continued hypnotic use. Perhaps most surprising is how little we know about each of these.

CHAPTER 9

Hypnotics and the Elderly

The effects of hypnotics in the elderly are of particular concern, because of their disproportionately high use of these agents and their increased vulnerability to toxicity from them. In 1975, 20–45% of prescriptions for the various hypnotics went to persons over 60 (Cooper, 1977), who comprised roughly 14% of the population. This is perhaps in keeping with the proportionately greater percentage of all prescriptions (roughly 20%) which the elderly receive (Subcommittee on Long Term Care, 1974).

As discussed in Chapter 2, population studies of reported usage of hypnotics also show an increase with age. A nationwide survey by the National Institute on Drug Abuse, for instance, indicated that 11% of persons over 50 reported they had taken a sedative defined as a hypnotic phenobarbital or butabarbital for medical use in the past year, compared to 6% of those 18–25 (Abelson *et al.*, 1977).*

The greater usage of hypnotics by the elderly takes on added significance in view of their increased susceptibility to adverse reactions to a variety of types of medications (Hurwitz, 1969; Pemberton, 1954; Seidl, Thornton, Smith, & Cluff, 1966). Hurwitz (1969), for instance, found that persons over 60 were 2.5 times more likely to experience drug reaction while in the hospital compared with those below this age. We will later discuss a variety of hypnotics—including some which generally are considered very benign—in which this age-related increase in toxicity is seen in population studies. This may result in hospitalizations which might otherwise have been prevented. In an Australian study, 16% of admis-

---

*The use of anxiolytics was also found to increase with age; stimulants, on the other hand, were most commonly used in the 26- to 34-year-old group.

sions to a geriatric psychiatry unit were found to be due to toxic reactions to psychoactive medication (about half of which were anxiolytics or hypnotics), which cleared when medications are discontinued (Learoyd, 1972). All of these problems are compounded by the increased number of medications taken by the elderly (11.4 prescriptions per year for persons over 65 compared to 4.0 for younger adults; Task Force on Prescription Drugs, 1969), which may make them more likely to experience undesirable interactions between drugs.

Before discussing the pharmacologic issues of hypnotic use in the elderly, which comprise the main focus of this section, it would be well to examine briefly the present patterns of such usage. One source of data on this area is a NIDA-sponsored study of 447 noninstitutionalized elderly subjects living in the Washington, D.C., area in 1976 (Guttmann, 1977). It was found that 62% of respondents were using prescription drugs daily, while 69% (the categories are not mutually exclusive) took over-the-counter (OTC) drugs. Of those taking prescription drugs, 13.6% were taking prescription anxiolytics or hypnotics daily (2.5% of those taking OTC drugs were taking OTC hypnotics). The sedative–hypnotics comprised the overwhelming majority of psychoactive drugs; the only other well-defined category was antidepressants, in 1.1% of respondents. Of those taking sedative–hypnotics as a whole, the pattern of usage was as follows: 40.5% daily; 40.5%, as needed; and 18.9% one or more times per week. There was also opportunity for interactions of medications with ethanol, as 38% reported regular use of either prescription or OTC drugs plus ethanol. Persons taking sedative–hypnotics tended to feel that they had unsatisfactory family relationships, to have more dissatisfaction with their lives, and yet felt that they had greater capabilities compared to those who did not use these agents. One suspects a great deal of human suffering beneath these objectively reported personality traits.

PHARMACOLOGY IN THE ELDERLY

Several recent reviews have described in detail the issues of pharmacology in the elderly (Bender, 1974; Hollister, 1977; Richey, 1975). One factor which alters the distribution of drugs in the elderly is the age-related changes in body composition. Fat may increase from 10% at age 20 to 24% at age 60. In principle, this might be expected to lead to increased storage of lipid-soluble drugs (Hollister, 1977), which is reflected in pharmacokinetic terms as a larger volume of distribution. Percentage of water, total body weight, and amounts of circulating plasma albumin may decrease. Since albumin is a major source of drug binding, its decrease might be expected to lead to greater amounts of free drug available to cross membranes and produce pharmacologic effects. It has also been suggested that there is altered central nervous system sensitivity in the elderly; in animal models, for instance, there is increased central sensitivity to catecholamines, insulin, camphor, and acetylcholine (Frolkis, Bezrukov, & Sinitsky, 1972). It has been suggested that this explains the proclivity for older patients to develop organic brain syndromes from relatively low doses of anticholinergic agents (Hollister, 1977). There are few data available on this point, however.

One relatively well-documented physiological change in the elderly is an altered pattern of absorption of drugs from the gastrointestinal tract. Studies of xylose and iron, which like most drugs are passively absorbed, show a decreased peak blood level, greater delay until the peak level, and prolonged rate of decay (Dietze, Kalbe, Kranz, Brusckke, & Richter, 1971; Guth, 1968) in patients over 80. It should be noted, however, that a slower rate of absorption is important in the timing of the initial action of a drug, but may have little to do with the amount of available effective drug when it is given chronically. In contrast to such agents as xylose and iron, there are unfortunately few data available on age-related changes in absorption of psychoactive drugs. Diazepam, however, has been studied in patients over 60, and shows the changes described above for xylose and iron (Garattini, Marcucci, Morselli, & Mussini, 1973). The decreased absorption may be related to a decrease in number of absorbing cells and blood flow (the latter may be decreased by 40–50% in patients over 65). Another complication resulting from decreased blood flow is that it does not affect the absorption of all drugs uniformly; animal studies suggest that those which are most lipid soluble are more sensitive to blood flow (Winne, 1971). Other physiological changes altering drug absorption in the elderly include decreased production of acid in the stomach and decreased gastrointestinal motility.

In addition to changes in absorption, the elderly may also have a decreased ability to metabolize and excrete some drugs. O'Malley, Crooks, Duke, and Stevenson (1971) showed significant increases in the plasma half-lives of antipyrine and phenylbutazone in the elderly, and attributed these changes to decreased drug metabolism. Direct measurement of a major metabolite of amobarbital, 3-hydroxyamobarbital, has demonstrated decreased formation in subjects over 65 compared to those 20–40 years of age. In animals, the data are inconsistent. Kato, Vassanelli, Frontino, and Chiesara (1964), and Trabucchi and Chiesara (1964), showed that in rats the microsomal activity responsible for metabolizing such drugs as meprobamate, pentobarbital, and hexobarbital is decreased. When Kato, Takanaka, and Onoda (1970) attempted to repeat these studies in mice, however, there were no clear age differences. There may also be sexual differences in rates of drug metabolism in the elderly, possibly due to the effects of gonadal hormones (or their lack) on liver function (O'Malley et al., 1971); Streicher & Garbus, 1955). A final complicating factor: because of the multiple mechanisms of metabolism, it is hazardous to generalize from the processing of one drug to how another will be metabolized. The rapidity with which a patient metabolizes antipyrine, for instance, is not predictive of his phenylbutazone metabolic rate (Richey, 1975).

Another aspect of liver function is, of course, biliary excretion of drugs and their metabolites. Tests of bromsulfalein (BSP) retention in the elderly have not been entirely consistent, but tend to suggest that there is no major impairment of BSP excretion with age (Calloway & Merrill, 1965; Koff, Garvey, Burney, & Bell, 1973).

In summary, evidence suggests that there may be a decrease in the ability of the liver to metabolize some drugs in the elderly, and probably little or no loss of biliary excretion. The data, however, are not as consistent as might be desired, and the clinical importance of changes in hepatic function in the elderly is not entirely clear. Hollister (1977) has concluded that there is little evidence to suggest that decreased liver function in the elderly is related to any specific clinical pharmacologic problem.

In contrast to hepatic excretion of drugs, renal excretion is clearly impaired in the elderly. This is largely related to decreased blood flow and glomerular filtration rate, which may be reduced by 45% in subjects over 65 compared to 25-year-old men (Holloway, 1974). This might be expected particularly to inhibit excretion of the more water-soluble drugs (and water-soluble metabolites of other drugs). Epidemiologically, renal impairment has in fact been correlated with incidence of adverse drug reactions (J.W. Smith, Seidl, & Cluff, 1966).

The various factors discussed here contribute to the longer half-lives of many drugs in the elderly. Klotz et al. (1975) and others, however, have cautioned that it should not be assumed that increased half-lives are due to decreased ability to metabolize and excrete drugs. In the case of diazepam, for instance, they found that there was no age-related decrease in clearance; rather, the prolonged half-life was due to an increased volume of distribution (see Chapter 3).

In summary, many of the physiologic changes of aging produce alterations in absorption, distribution, metabolism, and excretion of drugs. These changes plus possibly altered central nervous system sensitivity may help explain the high incidence of adverse drug reactions in the elderly.

EFFICACY STUDIES

Considering the widespread consumption of hypnotics by the elderly, it is striking how infrequently they have been used as subjects in efficacy studies. There are almost no EEG studies available; non-EEG studies are summarized in Table XII. It should be noted that with one exception (Reeves, 1977) virtually all these studies were done on inpatients. The scarcity of data precludes drawing any general conclusions as to the most effective hypnotic. Four studies in which barbiturates were compared with other agents found them superior to placebo in maintaining sleep (as reported by nursing observations) and usually similar to other hypnotics tested (Exton-Smith, 1963; Le Riche & Csima, 1964; Mellor & Imlah, 1966; Stotsky, Cole, Tang, & Gahm, 1971).

The two studies in which a high dose (200 mg amobarbital) was used indicated more side effects than other drugs (Exton-Smith, Hodkinson, & Crowie, 1963; Mellor & Imlah, 1966); the two studies in which more standard doses (50–100 mg butabarbital, 100 mg secobarbital) were used showed no more side effects than placebo (Stotsky *et al.*, 1971) or than other hypnotics (Le Riche & Csima, 1964). A comparison of 50 mg amobarbital and 15 mg flurazepam (with no placebo) for 14 nights found that patients reported roughly equal benefits in a global rating, and no significant side effects from either agent (Fisher & Gal, 1969). In a 1-month study, geriatric outpatients reported that both 0.25 mg triazolam and 15 mg flurazepam improved their sleep latency and "depth" of sleep, but only triazolam increased total sleep duration (Reeves, 1977). A 1-week study of 15 mg flurazepam, 60 mg fosazepam, and 5 mg nitrazepam showed only a nonsignificant trend for nurses' ratings of decreased awakenings with all drugs (Viukari *et al.*, 1978). They also noted increased awakenings during withdrawal from nitrazepam, in particular, which has been noted in other studies (see Chapter 4). A 2-week comparison of 25 mg thioridazine and 10 mg nitrazepam indicated that both drugs aided sleep induction but only thioridazine increased sleep duration (Linnoila & Viukari, 1976). The ability to conduct daytime affairs, as well as coordination, was found to be impaired by nitrazepam but not thioridazine. After administration for 5–21 nights, 250 mg glutethimide was considered more effective than placebo in an overall patient and staff rating which considered sleep induction and maintenance, and awakening refreshed (Asbell, 1962).

In sum, hypnotic efficacy studies in the elderly are comprised almost entirely of non-EEG studies of inpatient populations, in which no particular agent has been shown to be particularly advantageous. The next

TABLE XII. Efficacy Studies

Author	Subjects	Drugs
Linnoila & Viukari, 1976	20 geriatric psychiatry inpatients age 72 ± 6 (some received daytime haloperidol)	10 mg nitrazepam 25 mg thioridazine placebo
Viukari et al., 1978	17 geriatric psychiatry inpatients, usually with dementia, age 77 ± 2	15 mg flurazepam 60 mg fosazepam 5 mg nitrazepam placebo
Reeves, 1977	41 male and female geriatric outpatients complaining of insomnia	0.25 mg triazolam 15 mg flurazepam placebo
Pathy, 1975	47 geriatric nonpsychotic medical inpatients	384 mg chlormethiazole 443 mg dichloralphenazone placebo
F.H. Stern, 1972	43 nursing home patients, ages 66–87	Two tablets each containing 3 gr aspirin, 2.5 gr acetoaminophen, and 2 gr salicylamide in combination with either 25[a] or 36.5 mg methapyriline fumarate
Stotsky et al., 1971	53 male and female hospitalized psychiatric patients, ages 65–88; some patients on major tranquilizers during daytime.	50 and 100 mg butabarbital placebo

[a] Excedrin®.
[b] Mandrax®.

of Hypnotics in the Elderly

Method	Duration	Efficacy	Side effects
Nurses' ratings	14 nights	Sleep induction faster than placebo for both drugs; sleep duration greater than placebo with thioridazine but not nitrazepam.	Coordination, tapping speed, and ability to conduct daytime affairs decreased with nitrazepam but not thioridazine.
Nurses' ratings	7 nights	Nonsignificant trend for decreased number of awakenings and time spent awake with all drugs; on first withdrawal night there was an increased number of awakenings and time spent awake with nitrazepam compared to the last placebo night.	Strength of handgrip, coordination, short- and long-term memory not impaired in most patients; two patients with cerebrovascular disease became amnesic after all hypnotics.
Questionnaire	1 month	Triazolam superior to flurazepam on duration of sleep; both agents superior to placebo on various measures.	8 of 14 patients reported 17 side effects on triazolam; 6 of 13 patients reported 11 side effects on flurazepam; 1 of 14 patients on placebo reported side effects.
Patient ratings	7 nights	"Heavy sleep" more frequent with both drugs in comparison to placebo; heavy sleep and short sleep onset more frequent with chlormethiazole than dichloralphenazone.	Incidence of side effects on both drugs not distinguishable from placebo.
Nurses' observations and patient reports	1–3 night	Both medicines induced sleep more rapidly than placebo.	No increase in reported adverse effects compared to placebo.
Nurses' ratings	7 nights, each	Both doses equally effective and better than placebo; patients on 50 mg tended to improve in daytime behavior more than patients on placebo or 100 mg.	Confusion occurred in four patients on placebo, one on butabartal 50 mg, and two on butabarbital 100 mg.

Continued

TABLE XII

Author	Subjects	Drugs
Fisher & Gal, 1969	27 male geriatric inpatients, ages 60–88	15 mg flurazepam 50 mg amobarbital (no placebo)
Haider, 1968	48 geriatric psychiatry inpatients, ages 51–80	250 mg methaqualone plus 25 mg diphenlydramine[b] 650 mg dichloralphenazone (no placebo)
Kramer, 1967	35 male and female nursing home patients with OBS, ages 54–95	500 mg chloral hydrate 150 mg methaqualone (no placebo)
Mellor & Imlah, 1966	40 female geriatric psychiatry in-patients, ages 63–87 (receiving chlorpromazine by day)	200 mg amobarbital 500 mg glutethimide 500 mg ethchlorvynol placebo
Le Riche & Csima, 1964	25 male and female long-term-care patients, ages 47–97	500 mg ethchlorvynol 500 mg glutethimide 500 mg chloral hydrate 100 mg secobarbital placebo
Exton-Smith, 1963	65 female geriatrics patients, ages 59–63	200 mg amobarbital 1.3 gm dichloralphenazone 50 mg promazine resinate 800 mg meprobamate placebo
Asbell, 1962	38 male and female medical patients with insomnia	150 mg 2-methyl-3-0-tolyl-4-quinazolone (Hyptor®) 250 mg glutethimide placebo

[a] Excedrin-PM®.
[b] Mandrax®.

(Continued)

Method	Duration	Efficacy	Side effects
Patient interview	14 nights	For both drugs, patients stated they were sleeping as well or better than at previous times when they had used other hypnotics.	No significant side effects; no evidence of cumulative effect or habituation.
Nurses' observations, patient and staff preferences	3 nights	Patients and staff preferred Mandrax® to dichloralphenazone; sleep induction faster and duration longer with Mandrax® compared to dichloralphenazone.	
Psychiatric and nursing observations	14 nights	For both drugs patients stated they were sleeping "as well or better" than at previous times when they had used other hypnotics.	Three fourths of the patients on chloral hydrate had confusion and belligerence; no significant side effects on methaqualone.
Nurses' ratings	1 night	Patients were asleep at hourly observations significantly more frequently with ethchlorvynol and amobarbital, but not glutethimide.	Disturbed nighttime behavior and side effects more common with amobarbital than with placebo or other drugs.
Nurse reports	5 days	All medications induce sleep and better quality sleep than placebo, but not different from each other.	More drowsiness with glutethimide.
Patient questionnaire, nurse observations	1 night each	All drugs similar in maintaining sleep (number of hourly checks in which nurse found patient to be asleep), but meprobamate and dichloralphenazone preferred by patients.	Less drowsiness on dichloralphenazone and meprobamate.
Patient, nurse, and physician reports		Both equal and better than placebo in terms of an overall rating (going to sleep in less than 0.5 hr, sleeping 6 hr, awakening refreshed).	No significant side effects; no evidence of habituation.

consideration, then, should be the relative hazards of these agents in the elderly.

TOXICITY

Complications from psychopharmacologic agents in the elderly have been classified by Learoyd (1972) into three groups: (1) drug intoxication, including lethargy, confusion, and disorientation; (2) secondary drug effects such as hypotensive syncope and respiratory depression; and (3) disinhibition reactions, including restlessness and aggression. These "paradoxical reactions" to thioridazine have been related by some authors to certain personality traits (Slater & Kastenbaum, 1966). The occurrence of such reactions has often been associated with use of barbiturates (Gibson, 1966); it is important to note that they have been described with agents from all classes of hypnotics (Learoyd, 1972). In one study in which 25 elderly patients were each given four hypnotics (ethchlorvynol, glutethimide, chloral hydrate, and secobarbital), for instance, the barbiturate was the only agent that did not produce paradoxical excitement (Le Riche & Csima, 1964). A major problem is that such drug-induced restlessness is often misinterpreted as a sign of inadequate medication, and the dose is increased. Chloral hydrate, which is known for its relative paucity of side effects, has been reported by one group to be particularly troublesome in geriatric psychiatry patients. Kramer (1967) reported that of 19 patients with chronic brain syndromes who received 500 mg chloral hydrate, 14 developed confusion and hallucinations which cleared in 11 cases when medication was discontinued. Seven were subsequently given methaqualone without difficulty. Flurazepam, which is generally considered relatively benign, has an increasing incidence of toxicity with age (Greenblatt et al., 1977). In the Boston Collaborative (1972) study of hospitalized medical patients, 1.9% of patients under 60 years old had adverse reactions; this rose to 7.1% in patients over 80. Among patients 70 years or older taking the higher dose (30 mg) there were adverse reactions in 39%; with 15 mg this dropped to 2%. The most common difficulties were drowsiness, confusion, or ataxia. (Other data from this same study suggested that "clinical toxicity" from pentobarbital, secobarbital, and chloral hydrate does not increase with age.) Adverse effects of flurazepam in the elderly appeared somewhat more pronounced in a study of 195 nursing home patients. Marttila et al. (1977) reported that in this group 26% experienced toxic reactions to flurazepam, including ataxia, confusion, and hallucinations. Nitrazepam (10 mg) has also been reported to produce significant impairment of coordination and ability to conduct daily affairs in geriatric psychiatry patients (Linnoila & Viukari, 1976), although this seemed much less of a problem with 5 mg (Viukari *et al.*, 1978).

There is also an age-related increase in daytime drowsiness from some benzodiazepines. The Boston Collaborative Surveillance Program (1973) reported that among medical inpatients receiving diazepam and chlordiazepoxide as anxiolytics there was more drowsiness with advancing age, whereas this trend was not present with phenobarbital. Among patients 61–70 years old, drowsiness was slightly less with phenobarbital than the benzodiazepines (5.6% versus 8.6%) and in those over 70 the incidence was similar (12.1% versus 10.9%). In passing, it is interesting that cigarette smoking was correlated with less drowsiness from benzodiazepines, perhaps because cigarette smoke may stimulate hepatic drug-metabolizing enzymes. This effect did not occur with phenobarbital, perhaps because the barbiturate itself induces the enzymes.

Another potential problem has been raised by the observation in a retrospective study that blood calcium concentrations in elderly non-epileptic subjects were decreased in those receiving barbiturates compared to those on nitrazepam or diazepam (Young, Ramsay, & Murray, 1977). Whether this process (which may be related to alterations in vitamin D metabolism subsequent to hepatic enzyme induction) is actually manifest as an increased incidence of clinical osteomalacia is not yet known. The possibility should be borne in mind while awaiting more definitive data.

SUMMARY AND CONCLUSIONS

The elderly, who take a disproportionately high amount of hypnotics, are particularly vulnerable to toxic effects due to altered absorption, distribution, and clearance of drugs, possibly altered nervous system sensitivity, and the greater likelihood of receiving multiple drugs. These potential dangers are borne out by empirical data indicating an increased incidence of adverse reactions to medications in general and hypnotics in particular. It seems clear that one cannot predict incidence of a hypnotic's toxicity in the elderly from studies of young adults. There is tentative evidence, for instance, that flurazepam and chloral hydrate, which enjoy reputations for their lack of side effects, may both have substantially increased toxicity when used in elderly inpatients. On the other hand, daytime drowsiness from phenobarbital may not increase with age. Although case reports often point to the problem of confusional states with the barbiturates, these occur with all classes of sedative–hypnotics. Given the decreased efficiency of metabolism of many drugs in the elderly, the many benign features of the benzodiazepines must be weighed against their very long half-lives (50–100 hr for a major metabolite of flurazepam compared to approximately 24 hr for the hypnotic barbiturates). Any clinical significance which this difference in half-lives may have will undoubtedly be magnified in the elderly. These sorts of problems lead to the general impression that most data on efficacy and safety of hypnotics are derived from studies of younger adults, and their conclusions do not always apply to the elderly.

Data on hypnotic efficacy come predominantly from non-EEG studies of institutionalized subjects, who may not be representative of many elderly hypnotic users. The data which are available do not clearly indicate that one class of hypnotics is particularly more efficacious.

Clearly, it is desirable to use the least medicine possible in the elderly. Polypharmacy is to be discouraged, and doses of medication should be reduced when multiple medicines are given. This common-sense approach is apparently not practiced as widely as it might be. In one study of geriatric psychiatry patients, patients receiving multiple psychoactive drugs were usually on the same or higher doses than those receiving a single drug (Fracchia, Sheppard, Canale, Ruest, Cambria, & Merlis, 1975). One study of geriatric psychiatry patients showed that use of chloral hydrate could be reduced greatly by giving moderate amounts of wine (Mishara & Kastenbaum, 1974). Although ethanol has relatively little effect on total sleep time in animals and normal humans (Mendelson et al., 1977; Mendelson & Hill, 1978), it certainly decreases sleep latency markedly, and could reasonably be expected to aid in inducing a more rapid sleep onset. Dawson-Butterworth (1970) has demonstrated how careful assessment of hypnotic effects on inpatients can result in drastic reduction in their use. Certainly the use of conservative prescribing of hypnotics, which is important at all ages, is a first step in reducing toxicity in the elderly.

CHAPTER 10

Other Pharmacologic Approaches

Pharmacologic alternatives to prescription hypnotics include the over-the-counter (OTC) sleep aids, L-tryptophan, and ethanol. Perhaps the most striking thing about the OTC hypnotics is how little is known about them when one considers their widespread use. The effects of ethanol and L-tryptophan on sleep have been reviewed by a number of writers and will be briefly summarized here.

OVER-THE-COUNTER HYPNOTICS

There are perhaps 500,000 OTC medications with which Americans treat themselves for a variety of problems (Hecht, 1976), and for which they paid over $4 billion* in 1977 (Product Marketing, 1978a). Encouraged by substantial amounts of advertising† they have purchased over 30 million packages of OTC hypnotics annually since 1973 (Product Marketing, 1978a). In comparison, there were 26 million hypnotic prescriptions written in 1977 according to the National Prescription Audit; Institute of Medicine, 1979.) A survey conducted in 1971 found that OTC hypnotics had been used by 6% of men and women in the past year, compared to

---

*In contrast, retail sales for prescription drugs in 1977 were over $9 billion (Product Marketing, 1978a).

†Advertising expenditures in all media for headache remedies, sedatives, and sleeping preparations in 1977 were $123,033,200 (Product Marketing, 1978b).

3% and 4% who had taken prescription hypnotics (Balter & Bauer, 1975). (They also noted that users of OTC hypnotics may be a somewhat different population, tending to be younger, 18–44 years old, and more evenly balanced between the sexes than users of prescription hypnotics.) A general tendency among all OTC products is that a relatively small number of drugs are found in the large number of commercial preparations. It has been estimated, for instance, that only about 200 active medications are found in the approximately 500,000 available products (Hodes, 1974). This is very clearly the case among OTC hypnotics. A review of 41 of them found that 80% contained an antihistamine (usually methapyrilene) and 58% contained an anticholinergic (often scopolamine); as the figures indicate, many products are combination of the two agents (Greenblatt & Shader, 1977). A smaller proportion (22%) contained bromides.

Compounds Used in OTC Hypnotics

Methapyrilene

This is a member of the ethylenediamine class of antihistamines, which also includes pyrilamine. (The latter is the only other antihistamine marketed in OTC products specifically for use as a hypnotic and appears in roughly three products.) Antihistamines of this type are sometimes referred to as "H1 blockers" because they block actions of histamine on capillary permeability and on vascular and bronchial smooth muscle (as opposed to some other actions such as increasing gastric secretion). In general, they share a number of properties including local anesthetic qualities, ability to relax arterioles in man, and anticholinergic properties.

Methapyrilene was introduced in 1947, one year after the introduction of diphenhydramine (S.M. Feinberg & Bernstein, 1947). It was noted at that time that 19% of hay fever patients receiving 50–200 mg/day experienced sedation, to a degree thought to be less than that of diphenhydramine. Methapyrilene usually appears in OTC products as the hydrochloride or fumarate, in doses of 10–50 mg. Considering its wide use, it is striking how few data are available on it. A Medline search for all articles on its pharmacodynamics and toxicity from 1966–1978, for instance, detected only eight articles. Thus many comments on its pharmacology are usually based on generalizations about antihistamines as a group. In general, most antihistamines are readily absorbed from the gastrointestinal tract; clinical effects are thought to start in 15–30 min and to last 4–6 hr (Douglas, 1975). Relatively few data have been reported on the metabolism and excretion of methapyrilene. Another antihistamine of a different class, diphenhydramine, is largely metabolized in the liver, with little if any appearing unchanged in the urine. Most of a single dose is excreted as metabolites in the urine within 24 hr of ingestion. Data from animal studies suggest that some antihistamines may induce hepatic enzymes (Conney, Davison, Gastel, & Burns, 1960); it is conceivable that increased drug metabolism is the mechanism by which pretreatment of rats with the antihistamine chlorcyclizine produces decreased duration of pentobarbital anesthesia (Thompson, Dolowy, & Cole, 1959). In contrast, concomitant administration of anthhistamines may potentiate sedation from barbiturates. In animal studies, a number of antihistamines (but not pyrilamine) potentiate toxicity of exogenous norepinephrine, and it is conceivable that they might interact with clinical synpathomimetic agents (Jori, 1966). Anticholinergic properties, which they possess to varying degrees, may induce symptoms discussed in the section on scopolamine. Effects on the fetus and newborn need to be considered, insofar as OTC products are often taken by pregnant women. (In a study of 231 pregnant women in the Houston area in 1969–1975, 3 % were taking OTC sedatives; R.M. Hill, Craig, Chaney, Tennyson, & McCulley, 1977.) Meclizine consumed in the first trimester of pregnancy has been associated with cleft palate and limb deformities (Schenkel & Vorherr, 1974). Another area of concern is possible carcinogenicity, the evidence for which has been summarized in recent FDA reports ("Over-the-counter . . ," 1975, 1978).

Scopolamine

This is a belladonna alkaloid, possessing potent anticholinergic effects. Although scopolamine is sometimes considered more sedating than atropine, animal studies suggest that their nervous system effects are similar if correction is made for differing potencies (Meyers & Abreu, 1952). Scopolamine has usually been marketed in OTC hypnotics as the aminoxide hydrobromide in doses of 0.15–0.25 mg; it has been claimed that the slower conversion to the base compound accounts for a reputed lower toxicity, but this has not been well established. It is used medically for its anticholinergic properties and for sedation and amnesia prior to childbirth. It may occasionally produce euphoria and agitation prior to sedation, particularly at higher dosages. If given to a patient in pain without a concomitant analgesic, it may induce marked excitement.

Scopolamine salts are rapidly absorbed. Tentative data from two subjects suggest a half-life of roughly 2 hr (Bayne, Tao, & Crisologo, 1975). It is mostly metabolized, only 1% appearing unchanged in the urine.

Overdoses of scopolamine are rarely fatal in adults (patients have survived overdoses of 500 mg) but may lead to toxic psychoses which sometimes have been initially mistaken for schizophrenia (Baile, De-Paulo, & Schmidt, 1977). The elderly may be particularly susceptible to this (Chapter 9). Anticholinergic effects such as dry mouth, dilated pupils, acceleration of the heart rate, as well as toxic psychiatric manifestations may be potentiated by other drugs with anticholinergic properties, including the antihistamines often found in OTC hypnotics in combination with scopolamine. Scopolamine rapidly crosses the placenta and may cause tachycardia and circulatory failure in the fetus as well as prolongation of labor or inhibition of respiration in the newborn (Schenkel & Vorherr, 1974).

Bromides

These compounds were introduced into medicine in the 1840s for the treatment of syphilis and later for epilepsy. Interestingly, barbiturates were the agents which came to replace bromides as antiepileptic agents, and bromides came to be used mostly as anxiolytics or hypnotics. Although irritating to the gastrointestinal system, bromides are absorbed rapidly. They are mostly excreted by the kidneys, with a very long half-life of about 12 days. Since it takes at least a week to establish therapeutic blood levels, there is little hypnotic effect after a single dose. Another implication of the long half-life is, of course, that substantial accumulation may occur with repeated use. This may lead to chronic toxicity, the main problem associated with the use of bromides. (Acute overdose is rarely a problem, possibly because gastrointestinal irritation may lead to vomiting.) Chronic brominism produces an acne-like rash, delirium, hallucinations, tremors, and a positive Babinski sign. Bromides cross the placenta and may produce intoxication of the newborn, and there is some suspicion of teratogenicity in animals and humans (Harned, Hamilton, & Cole, 1944; Opitz, Grosse, & Haneberg, 1972).

Efficacy

Considering the widespread use of OTC hypnotics, the available data on efficacy is very slight and not very encouraging. In one study of medical inpatients (Straus, Eisenberg, & Gennis, 1955) subjective reports indicated that 50 mg methapyrilene was more effective than placebo in inducing and maintaining sleep, while another (Teutsch et al., 1975) found them indistinguishable. Sunshine (1974) and G.M. Smith, Coletta, McBride, and McPeek (1974) examined the effects of mixtures of 50 mg methapyrilene plus analgesics on patients with mild pain and trouble sleeping (medical and surgical inpatients and postpartum patients, respectively), and found that patients reported better quality sleep compared to placebo. Wolff (1974) administered two Excedrin P.M. tablets (a mixture of 25 mg methapyrilene plus analgesics in each) for 2 weeks to self-described insomniacs; subjective reports indicated that the medication "helped" more, and induced sleep better than placebo. Similarly, F.H. Stern (1972) found that two Excedrin P.M. tablets given for 1 night to geriatric inpatients induced sleep (as judged by nurses' observations) more rapidly than placebo. Sleep maintenance was not improved in the Wolff study, and was not assessed by Stern. Inferences regarding the efficacy of metapyrilene must be tempered with the consideration that the analgesic-induced relief from pain in the inpatients may have aided sleep, and that aspirin itself (found in these compounds) may have some hypnotic properties (Hauri & Silberfarb, 1978). J. Kales, Tan, Swearingen, and Kales (1971) administered two Sominex tablets (25 mg methapyrilene and 0.25 mg scopolamine hydrobromide each) for 3 nights to five volunteers who complained of poor sleep and found no improvement in EEG sleep measures.

Federal Regulation

We are in a situation in which a group of drugs, for which there is little evidence of efficacy and some reason to suspect potential harm, is consumed in greater quantities than are prescription hypnotics. The economic incentives to market such agents are clear; until recently, the constraints on their manufacture and sale have been slight. It is worthwhile to discuss briefly the history of federal concern and authority in this area. The interested reader will find more detailed evaluations in reviews (Hodes, 1974; Moxley, Yingling, & Edwards, 1973) and FDA documents ("Over-the-counter . . ," 1975, 1978).

The first time that the federal government entered the area of drug regulation was with the Food and Drug Act of 1906, which required that drugs in interstate commerce meet their advertised standards of strength and purity. The Shirley Amendment to this act in 1912 further restricted fraudulent claims of therapeutic benefit. Following a tragedy in which over 100 persons died from poisoning by a particular preparation of sulfanilimide, Congress passed the Food, Drug and Cosmetic Act of 1938, which is the fundamental law under which the FDA operates. One of its outstanding features was that manufacturers were required to file an application with the FDA demonstrating that a new drug was safe if taken as recommended. The Wheeler–Lea Amendment to the Federal Trade Commission Act of the same year tightened restrictions on false advertising. The distinction between prescription and OTC drugs was made in the Durham–Humphrey Amendment to the Food, Drug and Cosmetic Act in 1952. It should be noted that in all this time, safety rather than efficacy was the primary focus of federal concern. It was not until 1962 that the Kefauver–Harris Amendments to the Food, Drug and Cosmetic Act required that a drug marketed since 1938 be shown to be efficacious as well as safe. One consequence of these amendments was that in 1966 the FDA requested the National Academy of Sciences/National Research Council to review the efficacy of available prescription and nonprescription drugs. In the course of this tremendous task, the NAS/NRC examined approximately 480 OTC drugs and concluded that about 15% were effective (in addition, 27% were probably effective, 47% possibly effective, and 11% ineffective). In the light of these findings, the FDA formulated a new method to help insure safety and efficacy of OTC products. In this plan the FDA would convene a series of panels of outside experts to review various classes of OTC drugs. These panels would produce monographs that would specify which ingredients may be found in drugs marketed for particular medical complaints, and which claims can be made for them. Manufacturers whose products and advertising conform to these standards would not need further FDA approval. Products deviating from these standards would have to be cleared by a New Drug Application to the FDA.

A panel on sleep aids, daytime sedatives, and stimulants began work in November 1972, and published its recommendations in 1975 ("Over-the-counter . . ," 1975). A tentative set of FDA orders based on this report, with subsequent modifications by the FDA, was published in 1978 ("Over-the-counter . . ," 1978), and at the time of this writing awaits final approval. Methapyrilene fumarate and hydrochloride were originally considered by the panel to be safe and effective; subsequent data raising the possibility of carcinogenicity led the FDA to suggest that these be placed in their category II (not generally considered safe or effective, or misbranded), which means that they would be taken off the market. The same fate was suggested for scopolamine hydrobromide or aminoxide hydrobromide because they were considered ineffective at the low doses employed in OTC hypnotics and unacceptably toxic at higher doses. It was suggested that bromides be removed from the market because the therapeutic dose is unacceptably close to the toxic range, and because of the potential for teratogenic effects. Three antihistamines which have not been used in OTC hypnotics—doxylamine succinate, phenyltoloxamine dihydrogen citrate, and diphenhydramine hydrochloride—were considered to be potentially marketable in the future if further studies find them to be safe and effective. (It should be noted that diphenhydramine, as a prescription drug, is often given to aid sleep.) Perhaps most important, pyrilamine maleate was considered to be in category III (meaning that insufficient data are available for a final classification), so that this agent may be marketed under the proviso that manufacturers have 3 years in which to provide data that it is safe and effective.

L-TRYPTOPHAN

L-tryptophan is an essential amino acid, consumed in a normal diet in quantities of 0.5–2.0 grams per day. Although not marketed as a hypnotic, it is available in health food stores in the United States, and is used as an antidepressant in Great Britain. Hartmann (1978) has recently summarized 11 trypotophan studies from his laboratory (one with rats and ten with normal human volunteers and mild insomniacs) in most of which doses as little as 1.0 gm reduced sleep latency. A review of ten human studies (which included normals, insomniacs, narcoleptics, and schizophrenics) from several laboratories found that four reported increased total sleep time while four reported no change (Mendelson *et al.*, 1977). A number of reports have indicated that slow-wave sleep is increased; reports on REM sleep have been variable.

Although it has sometimes been suggested that the effects of L-tryptophan on sleep are due to its conversion to serotonin, it is important to bear in mind that this is only one of its metabolic routes. It may be converted to tryptamine and ultimately indoleacetic acid, or may follow a pathway to kynurenine and its products. One human study seems to indicate that its effects on sleep are not due to increases in serotonin (Wyatt, 1972). When L-tryptophan was administered to patients in whom serotonin synthesis was partially inhibited by pretreatment with parachlorophenylalanine, it still had pronounced effects on sleep (increased nonREM and decreased REM sleep).

Although a number of people have used L-tryptophan in the last 15 years, there are no documented cases of serious abuse or suicide. Side effects are generally uncommon, except perhaps for nausea, which is more often associated with doses above the usual recommended hypnotic range of 1–5 gm. The attractions of L-tryptophan await confirmation in well-defined chronic insomniacs, particularly in comparison with more traditional hypnotics. Little is known about long-term effects, which conceivably could include alterations in protein synthesis. There is some tentative evidence linking tryptophan metabolites to bladder cancer in animals (Bryan, 1971), a possibility which must be studied further before recommending its more widespread use.

ETHANOL

Ethanol is, of course, widely used by itself and in combination with hypnotics (Chapter 7) to aid sleep. In a survey of 549 self-described insomniacs in Los Angeles, it was the single most commonly used drug at the time of questioning, although it was taken less frequently than all prescription and OTC medicines combined (Guilleminault et al., 1977). The effects of ethanol on sleep have recently been reviewed in detail (Mendelson, 1979). In animals and normal humans, its hypnotic effects are manifested primarily by reducing sleep latency rather than by increasing total sleep. REM sleep may be decreased and slow-wave sleep increased, even when bedtime blood ethanol concentrations are below those which would produce inerbiation (Yules, Lippman, & Freedman, 1967). The relative lack of effect on total sleep presumably reflects its rapid metabolism, which proceeds in a linear manner at a rate of roughly 10–20 mg percent per hour during both waking and sleeping (Knowles et al., 1968; Williams & Salamy, 1972). E.P. Hurd, a Massachusetts physician writing in 1891, described his experiences giving ethanol to insomniacs:

> Unfortunately, the sleep produced by alcohol is often of short duration; the patient awakes after a couple of hours but little refreshed, and may be awake much of the night without being able to go to sleep again. (p. 94)

Although this may somewhat exaggerate the late-night increase in restlessness which may be associated with ethanol in nonalcoholic subjects, it does suggest a short-lived effect. Similarly, the insomniacs in the Los Angeles study (Guilleminault et al., 1977) reported three to one that ethanol aided sleep induction but were evenly divided as to whether it helped maintain sleep. There is some laboratory evidence that motor restlessness is increased late at night (Mullin et al., 1933).

Chronic alcoholics have persistent sleep EEG changes including increased REM sleep, number of arousals, and changes in sleep stages, as well as decreased slow-wave sleep (Lester, Rundell, Cowden, & Williams, 1973). The latter may be observed for 1 to 2 years (Adamson & Burdick, 1973) or even 4 years (Wagman & Allen, 1974) after cessation of drinking. When alcoholics drink, there may be decreased REM and increased slow-wave sleep. Discontinuing ethanol is often, but not always (Johnson, Burdick, & Smith, 1970), followed by decreased total sleep (Allen, Wagman, Faillace, & McIntosh, 1971; Gross, Goodenough, Hastey, & Lewis, 1973; Greenberg & Pearlman, 1967; Gross, Goodenough, Tobin, Halpert, Lepose, Perlstein, Sirota, Dibianco, Fuller, & Kishmer, 1966). Usually after several nights there is a large increase in REM sleep; in those patients who experience delirium tremens, this may be so exaggerated that it comes to represent over 90% of sleep time (Greenberg &

Pearlman, 1967; Gross, Goodenough, Hastey, & Lewis, 1973; Johnson *et al.*, 1970). Some of the implications of the REM rebound to the process of dependence have been discussed in Chapter 8.

Although there is a great deal of data on the effects of ethanol on the sleep EEG of control subjects and alcoholics, there are relatively few systematic data on its usefulness as a sleep aid when given in moderation to insomniacs. In view of its relatively short action and dependence-prone nature, it is not clear how widely its use should be recommended. It is interesting that in the controlled conditions of a geriatric psychiatry ward the availability of wine resulted in decreased consumption of chloral hydrate (Mishara & Kastenbaum, 1974).

SUMMARY AND CONCLUSIONS

OTC hypnotics are taken extensively, probably more often than prescription hypnotics. There is some evidence that the populations taking OTC and prescription hypnotics may be somewhat different, with OTC users tending to be somewhat younger and to be more equally balanced between the sexes. The most common ingredients in these products are methapyrilene and scopolamine salts (alone or in combination) and bromides. There are very few data on efficacy of these compounds, and they show results which are mixed. All of these agents present issues of toxicity, and methapyrilene may possibly be carcinogenic. For these reasons, it is likely that they may be withdrawn from the market in the near future.* Pyrilamine, structurally related to methapyrilene, will remain on the market while further testing is done, and the way has been left open for three other antihistamines to be tested for possible approval later. Given the tremendous investment in and sales of these agents, it takes little imagination to predict that manufacturers will tend to market OTC products containing pyrilamine or other agents. This is a situation which should be followed carefully.

There has been much interest in L-tryptophan as a hypnotic, and a number of animal and human studies have reported fairly consistently that it reduces sleep latency. There are few data available on efficacy in comparison to traditional hypnotics. An issue of possible carcinogenicity in animals has also been raised and needs further work. Ethanol is widely used to aid sleep induction, but is probably of little help in maintenance of sleep. Its use in controlled conditions has been recommended as an aid to sleep for the elderly.

*Note added in proof: On June 8, 1978, Health, Education, and Welfare Secretary Joseph A. Califano and an industry group, the Proprietary Association, announced a voluntary recall of most drugs containing methapyrilene, due to reports of carcinogenicity.

CHAPTER 11

Nonpharmacologic Treatment of Insomnia

The decision of whether to prescribe a hypnotic should include a consideration of alternative approaches. These consist primarily of counseling or psychotherapy, and of behavioral therapies. It might be well, then, to mention briefly the benefits available from each of these.

COUNSELING AND PSYCHOTHERAPY

Many physicians believe that office counseling is useful in treating insomnia. Attention may be directed to discomfort of accompanying medical illnesses, dealing with difficult situations, drinking, and so on. There are a number of suggestions falling into the realm of "sleep hygiene" which have not been tested empirically but which intuitively seem helpful. These include encouraging the patient to make his sleep hours regular, avoid daytime naps, not drink coffee or other stimulants at night, avoid tension-producing activities late at night. One can inquire about the comfort of the bed, noise and temperature in the bedroom, and whether there is a sense of physical security. Such counseling may not only be intrinsically useful, but may also serve as a vehicle for establishing the "helping" relationship which is important to the practice of good medicine.

Some authors have suggested that psychotherapy (sometimes with brief pharmacotherapy in addition) should be the major approach to treating most chronic insomniacs (A. Kales, Kales, & Humphrey, 1975).

An implication of this view is that insomnia represents a concrete "somatic" complaint which can otherwise prevent recognition of more profound psychological disturbances. This view gains strength from the several reports of abnormal MMPI scores in groups of insomniacs (Chapter 1). There are very few systematic data, however, on the utility of psychotherapy for this purpose. A recent exhaustive review of psychotherapy studies, for instance, has virtually no mention of insomnia (Parloff, Wolfe, Hadley, & Waskow, 1978).

BEHAVIORAL THERAPIES

General Considerations

A common theme in this heterogeneous group of treatments is an emphasis on altering objective behaviors, in contrast to subjective feelings which are the center of interest in psychoanalytically oriented therapy. The theories on which these methods are based are largely derived from studies of the experimental psychology of learning; they were stimulated by such authors as H.J. Eysenck, who argued that the principles of behavioral psychology might profitably be used to treat clinical disturbances.

Behavioral approaches to insomnia, which have recently been reviewed (Bootzin, 1977; Ribordy & Denney, 1977; Thoresen, Coates, Zarcone, Kirmil-Gray, & Rosekind, in press) might be arbitrarily classified as follows:

1. Relaxation based
   a. Biofeedback
   b. Progressive relaxation
   c. Autogenic training
   d. Meditation
2. Conditioning techniques
   a. Systematic desensitization
   b. Stimulus control
   c. Classical conditioning
3. Attribution therapy
4. Behavioral self-management

As pointed out by Ribordy and Denney (1977) and other authors, many of these techniques (relaxation, systematic desensitization, attribution-based therapies) are based on the hypothesis that poor sleep results from anxiety and an enhanced state of arousal, as manifested by increased autonomic activity such as heart rate, temperature, and vasoconstriction. This concept derives from the germinal study by Monroe (1967), which might be summarized as follows:

Monroe had subjects responding to bulletin board and newspaper ads fill out a questionnaire about their sleep habits. From these he selected 16 good and 16 poor sleepers. It is important to note, as Monroe did, that the poor sleepers did not have extremely disturbed sleep; none of them perceived themselves as "being insomniacs" or as suffering from a specific sleep disturbance. When he examined these groups, however, a variety of differences in physiological measures were found. Immediately before going to sleep, the poor sleepers had higher mean rectal temperature, heart rate, and phasic vasoconstriction rate. During sleep, they had higher temperature, phasic vasoconstrictions, body movements, and basal skin resistance.* The sleep EEG showed that the poor sleepers had less sleep time, a larger sleep latency, less REM, more awakenings, and more Stage 2. They also had more pathological scores on the Minnesota Multiphasic Personality Inventory (MMPI) and the Cornell Medical Index. Monroe took these findings to mean that "self-reported poor sleepers not only sleep less, but the sleep they obtain is more 'awake-like' than that of good sleeprs" (p. 263). This concept was thought to be supported by the finding by Johns, Gay, Masterton, and Bruce (1971) of higher 24-hour urinary 11-hydroxycorticosteroids in questionnaire-defined poor sleepers. On the other hand, frontalis muscle tension, which is thought to reflect manifest anxiety, has not been found to relate significantly to subjective sleep latency in 101 introductory psychology students (Haynes, Follingstad, & McGowan, 1974), although it did relate to a report of sleeping difficulties and number of times awake. Neither frontalis muscle tension (Good, 1975) nor EMG or heart rate (Freedman & Papsdorf, 1976) showed significant relations to EEG sleep latency in volunteers with varying sleep habits, and in self-reported insomniacs, respectively. In a study in which severe insomniacs were taught relaxation techniques, pre- and posttraining difference scores of cardiac rate, respiration, and skin conductance did not correlate with subjective evaluations of sleep (Lick & Heffler, 1977). In a study of EMG biofeedback with sleep-onset insomniacs, the treatment decreased frontalis muscle tension without significantly improving subjective or EEG sleep measures (Frankel, Coursey, Gaarder, & Mott, 1975). Similarly, pre- and posttreatment EMG or heart rate difference scores were not associated with subjective improvement in a study of progressive and hypnotic relaxation procedures (Borkovec &

---

*Monroe also noted that temperature, in the good sleepers, began to increase after 6:00–7:00 A.M., while this was not true of the poor sleepers. Another way to view the increased presleep temperature and lack of increase the next morning among the poor sleepers is that they may have had altered circadian processes (see Table I).

Fowles, 1973). Thus the notion that increased autonomic activity and skeletal muscle tension are important in the etiology of insomnia was derived from data on questionnaire-defined poor sleepers (not necessarily insomniacs who might be more typical of those who seek help), and has not stood up well in subsequent studies. It did, however, stimulate the performance of a variety of studies in which investigators attempted to improve sleep by enhancing presleep relaxation.

Relaxation Procedures

A major method which has been employed to induce relaxation has been electromyographic (EMG) biofeedback. In this procedure, electrodes are attached over muscle groups (often on the forehead), and the recorded muscle tension is transduced to sounds which vary with the degree of tension. The subject practices increasing the occurrence of the sound associated with reduced muscle tension. Other variants employed with insomniacs include EEG biofeedback in which the subject learns to maximize alpha (8.0–14.0 Hz) or theta (4.0–7.0 Hz) activity or "sensorimotor spindle rhythms" (13.5 Hz). Early published case histories of EMG biofeedback treatment of insomnia (e.g., Budzynski, Stoyva, & Adler, 1970) seemed promising, as did an uncontrolled study of patients with anxiety and insomnia and long-standing hypnotic use (Raskin, Johnson, & Rondestvedt, 1973). Budzynski (1973) reported the clinical impression that EMG biofeedback alone may be less useful to sleep-onset insomniacs than a combination of EMG and theta biofeedback.

Studies of other forms of relaxation training suffer many of the difficulties of the EMG studies. Among the earliest was a study of Kahn, Baker, and Weiss (1968), in which college students with disturbed sleep underwent four sessions of autogenic training plus home practice. (This method, developed by Schultz & Luthe, 1959, involves asking subjects repetitively to say a number of standard phrases involving a feeling of peacefulness and relaxation of the limbs.) Eleven of 13 subjects retrospectively considered their sleep to be improved, and the subjective reports of sleep latencies were shortened in each of the 10 patients in whom this was examined. There was, however, no independent control group; and there were no corroborating physiological measures.

Another form of relaxation training, referred to as progressive relaxation, is derived from the work of Jacobson (1938) and involves the systematic tensing and relaxing of specific muscle groups. Jacobson (1964) cited a number of cases in which he believed patients with insomnia to be benefited by this approach. Borkovec and Fowles (1973) compared progressive relaxation, hypnotic and self-relaxation procedures, and no treatment in introductory psychology students who reported sleep latencies greater than 45 min on a questionnaire. Although at 1 week after treatment the progressive relaxation and hypnosis groups improved more than the untreated subjects in terms of subjective sleep latency and feeling rested, there was equally good improvement in the self-relaxation group. This observation led the authors to discount the role of relaxation in the improvement and to consider the possibility of nonspecific factors. Among these were the focusing of attention on pleasant internal feelings, possibly precluding the continual ruminations characteristic of insomnia. Nicassio and Bootzin (1974) compared progressive relaxation, autogenic training, self-relaxation, and no treatment in volunteers who reported subjective sleep latencies with a mean of 120 min. They found that progressive relaxation and autogenic training produced significant and roughly equal subjective improvement in time to fall asleep (but not in total amount or quality of sleep) in comparison to the self-relaxation and untreated groups. As a 6-month follow-up these benefits were maintained in terms of subjective sleep latency but not for global improvement. The lack of efficacy of the self-relaxation group (in contrast to the findings of Borkovec and Fowles) were attributed to the less severely disturbed sleep in subjects in the latter study. The findings of Nicassio and Bootzin (1974) were essentially replicated by Lick and Heffler (1977), who used progressive relaxation procedures with and without an additional relaxation training tape recording, and compared these with an untreated group and a placebo group receiving modified "T-scope therapy" (in which autonomic arousal is paired with mild electrical shocks to the finger). Subjects were obtained from newspaper ads for insomniacs and complained of symptoms for approximately 11 years. Although the individual relaxation procedures did not improve subjectively reported sleep, there were improvements when the two treatment groups were combined and compared to the two control groups. (Results were reported for the period 30–50 days after the end of the treatment.) One interesting feature of this study was that the authors also examined the effects of treatment on use of hypnotics in 13 of the subjects who took them more than 25% of the time in the pretreatment period. A comparison of the 20 days before and after treatment indicated that either relaxation procedure significantly decreased hypnotic administration compared to the untreated group, although not when compared to the placebo treatment group. When the relaxation treatment groups were combined as before, however, hypnotic administration was significantly reduced compared to both the untreated and the placebo treatment group. As mentioned earlier, they found no relation between difference scores for physiologic variables and subjectively reported outcome. This led the authors to conclude that whereas relaxation procedures may be beneficial to severe insomniacs, their effects may not be mediated by a reduction in autonomic arousal.

One of the more comprehensive evaluations of the utility of relaxation procedures comes from the combined analysis of the three carefully performed studies (Freedman, Hauri, Coursey, & Frankel, 1978). The individual studies might be summarized as follows: Freedman and Papsdorf (1976) used advertisements to gather 18 persons with subjective difficulty in falling asleep for at least 6 months, and treated them with EMG biofeedback, progressive relaxation, or a control exercise procedure. Following a course of 6 half-hour training sessions there was a significant and approximately equal decrease in EEG sleep latency in the two experimental groups. Frankel et al. (1975) compared the effects of 6-week courses of EMG biofeedback, autogenic training, and electrosleep control treatment on 22 medically referred insomniacs with symptoms of at least 2 years' duration. (They had previously reported electrosleep to be ineffective, and considered it a control manipulation.) Although there was subjective and EEG improvement in approximately half of the patients in the EMG biofeedback and autogenic training groups over a 1-month follow-up period, neither group as a whole showed statistically significant improvement relative to the electrosleep control group. Hauri and Cohen (1977) treated medically referred insomniacs with symptoms of over 2 years' duration with three kinds of biofeedback (EMG, EMG plus theta, and SMR) and compared them to a group receiving "best medical treatment" without biofeedback. There were modest improvements in subjective sleep latency and EEG-determined sleep efficiency with EMG and SMR biofeedback, and virtually no change in the EMG plus theta biofeedback or untreated groups.

When these authors pooled their data (Freedman et al., 1978), they first covaried for age, since Freedman's college student population was significantly younger than all the other groups except Hauri's medical controls, but the results were unchanged. There were no differences between the groups in terms of MMPI scores or types of insomnia when classified into three general groups (sleep onset, intermittent waking, or no EEG changes). It was found that those patients who did improve (in terms of sleep latency and total time awake) tended to have had greater initial sleep latencies and total time awake and less Stage 2, and they were more often women. When the treatment groups were combined into biofeedback (EMG and EMG plus theta), relaxation (progressive relaxation and autogenic training), or control (electrosleep and exercise), there were no significant differences in improvement. The authors concluded, then, that while biofeedback and relaxation procedures may be effective with some patients, they are not recommended for insomniacs as a whole, and indicated the need for research into more effective treatments.

One possible means by which the efficacy of biofeedback might be improved would be if the type of biofeedback employed were tailored to the symptoms of the individual patient. Hauri and Cohen (1977) who, as described above, found limited improvement when EMG, EMG plus theta, and SMR feedback were assigned randomly to patients, examined this approach. They found that some of their patients seemed very tense and hypothesized that they were best treated with EMG biofeedback. Others seemed relaxed but had many awakenings, a large amount of Stage 1, or poor spindling; it was speculated that these might most appropriately be treated with SMR training. When they analyzed their data according to whether the randomly assigned patients had received the "appropriate" therapy, they found that the "appropriately" treated group had significant improvements in EEG sleep latency and sleep efficiency, while the group receiving "inappropriate" treatments did not. Thus it may be that when biofeedback, and possibly other relaxation therapies, are tailored to specific symptoms of insomnia, the previously gloomy results may improve.

Conditioning-Derived Therapies

In systematic desensitization procedures for insomnia, the patient is trained in a relaxation procedure such as progressive relaxation, and then the sensation of feeling relaxed is paired with images of going to bed. Case reports (e.g., Geer & Katkin, 1966) and essentially uncontrolled treatment studies (Borkovec, Steinmark, & Nau, 1973; Hinkle & Lutker, 1972) indicated that this might be of some benefit. Steinmark and Borkovec (1974) performed a controlled treatment study of college students with subjective sleep latencies greater than 30 min. Subjects were divided into four groups which parsed out the possible effects of the relaxation training alone: progressive relaxation, relaxation plus desensitization, quasi-desensitization control, and untreated patients. Treatments were given once a week for 4 weeks. In order to minimize the effects of expectation, subjects were told that no benefits were to be expected until after 4 weeks of treatment. During the first 3 weeks when this counter-demand principle was in effect, the subjective sleep latency of the two treatment groups improved equally, to a degree significantly better than the control groups. After the fourth week the quasi-desensitization control also improved compared to the untreated group, but this benefit was temporary; during a 5-month follow-up the sleep latencies in the two treatment groups continued to decrease, while those in the quasi-desensitization group became longer. Since the group which received progressive relaxation alone improved as much as the desensitization group, however, the benefits of desensitization *per se* in treating subjects with long sleep latencies were called into question.

Another conditioning-derived therapy which, like systematic desensitization, is based on operant conditioning principles, is the stimulus control technique. In this view, the act of falling asleep is considered an instrumental act which is performed in order to produce sleep, which is the reinforcer (Bootzin, 1977). The environment of the bedroom contains the discriminative stimuli, and insomnia results when these stimuli evoke behaviors other than falling asleep (e.g., worrying, watching TV, eating). The patient is instructed to associate the bedroom stimuli only with sleep. Thus he is told to lie down only if he is sleepy and to leave the bedroom if he is engaged in any activity other than sleep or sex. After success with an intensively studied case (Bootzin, 1972), a study was performed in which 78 subjects were divided into four groups, receiving stimulus control instuctions, progressive relaxation training, self-relaxation procedures, and no treatment (Bootzin, 1973, 1977). After 4 weeks of therapy, subjects receiving stimulus control instructions or progressive relaxation (whose pretreatment subjective sleep latency was about 90 min) had reductions by 74 and 38 min, respectively, which was a significantly greater decrease than in the other two conditions. They also reported a mean of 1 hr more sleep a night than the other groups, and the stimulus control subjects considered themselves to feel better upon awakening than those in other groups. A subsequent stimulus control study by Tokarz and Lawrence (1974) was positive, as was an unpublished study of Salma (cited by Bootzin, 1974) in which a counterdemand strategy was used—there was improvement even though subjects were told that the procedure would probably not help them. Haynes, Price, and Simons (1975), in a careful study of four self-described insomniacs with symptoms of several years' duration, examined stimulus control procedures in a study with an A–B–A–B design. Following a baseline period, subjects were instructed in stimulus control techniques; later, in a reversal period they returned to their former habits, and then once again applied the stimulus control rules. All four improved on a variety of subjective measures including sleep latency and daytime fatigue, although two did not get worse during the reversal phase. All four remained improved at a 9-month follow-up.

In contrast to the operant approaches that have been described above, classical conditioning techniques have been employed to induce sleep. Beilin (1952) in the Soviet Union reported increasing behavioral sleep in over 200 patients by pairing the use of sedative drugs (unconditioned stimulus) to heat, light, or sounds (conditioned stimuli). Marchand (1954) conditioned 20 patients to sleep after pairing hypnotic suggestion with a buzzer, although the relative roles of the conditioning and the effects of suggestion were unclear. Poser, Fenton, and Scotton (1965) treated a patient with a long history of anxiety, phobias, and hyposomnia by playing a metronome while injecting methohexital and then having the patient listen to a metronome at bedtime. Although there was no evidence of conditioning EEG sleep during daytime rest trials in which saline was injected while the metronome played, the patient found that the metronome was useful in inducing sleep or relaxation at home, and improved clinically. He remained better at follow-up several months later. Evans and Bond (1969) described treating a man who had suffered from insomnia since an automobile accident seven years previously, and who was unresponsive to systematic desensitization by reciprocal inhibition. In this case methohexital was injected while the patient counted from 1 to 28, although it is not clear if he was asked to practice counting at bedtime. The patient reported an increase in number of hours of sleep and fewer interruptions of sleep.

In sum, there have been several promising reports of using classical conditioning to improve insomnia, although this method awaits reconfirmation with new systematic, controlled studies.

Attributional Therapy

This approach is based on the work of such authors as Kelley (1967) and Heider (1958), who emphasized the importance of a subject's understanding of the causes of the psychological phenomena he experiences. Ross, Rodin, and Zimbardo (1969) performed a study which suggested to them that the manipulation of a subject's perception of the cause of arousal might have therapeutic benefits. Subjects were given a learning task, and were told that poor performance would be punished with an electric shock, the discomfort of which was emphasized. When one group was told that their heightened arousal (due to fear of shock) was actually related to loud background noises, the fearfulness decreased compared to subjects who attributed their stimulated state to their own fear. Storms and Nisbett (1970) explored this approach as a treatment for the presumed increase of arousal in insomniacs. The basic assumption was that attribution of arousal to an external source (i.e., a pill) might lead to decreased arousal. College students who answered advertisements for insomniacs were divided into three groups. One was given a placebo which they were told would enhance their arousal. The authors speculated that instead of increasing sleep latency due to suggestion, the pill would actually decrease sleep latency, as the subjects would view it as an emotionally neutral external force while they themselves experienced less emotion. Another group was told that the placebo pill would relax them. In this case, the authors hypothesized that the experience of difficulty falling asleep even when taking a sedative would be disturbing and hence make the insomnia worse. A third group received no pills. In both cases the authors' predictions were confirmed in terms of subjective sleep; i.e., the arousal condition patients reported shorter sleep latencies, while the relaxation patients reported an increase in time to fall asleep. On the other hand, the reported amount of suffering was not closely related to sleep latency—the arousal subjects said that their overall discomfort increased slightly, while it decreased in the relaxation group. Thus the results of this particular attribution process may have been more useful as a stimulus to further studies and new approaches than a therapeutic tool. This study has also suffered difficulty in replication. Kellogg and Baron (1975) found essentially the opposite of what might have been predicted by Storms and Nisbett (1970). Subjects who were told that the medication had stimulating effects did in fact have prolonged subjective sleep latencies. In a study by Bootzin, Herman, and Nicassio (1976) the results of Storms and Nisbett (1970) also failed to be replicated. Subjects who were told that their (placebo) pill would stimulate them were not affected, while those who were told that the pill would relax them did in fact report falling asleep faster. An unpublished study by Lowery, Denney, and Storms (1976, cited by Ribordy & Denney, 1977) failed to confirm any effects on subjective sleep latency, but did suggest that these manipulations might lessen the sense of difficulty in falling asleep. Given this variety of outcomes, it seems unlikely that this particular form of source reattribution is of any usefulness. One tantalizing thought comes from the Lowery, Denney, and Storms (unpublished manuscript, 1976) study, however. An additional experimental group was told that their light sleep should be attributed to a nonpejorative characteristic about themselves—that they tended to have relatively high levels of physiologic arousal. This was reported to result in decreased difficulty in falling asleep.

Another variation in attribution therapy is to hypothesize that improvement will occur if the subject can attribute to himself the ability to fall asleep easily. Thus, Davidson, Tsujimoto, and Glaros (1973) performed a study on "subjects complaining of insomnia" who were given a treatment program consisting of a combination of 1000 mg chloral hydrate, relaxation training, and instructions in practical sleep hygiene such as making their bedtimes very consistent. Those who improved after a week were divided into two groups. One was told that they were receiving a generally effective dosage of medication and thus that their improvement was derived from an external source. The other was told that they had been given a minimally effective dose, and hence that their improvement might be ascribed to their own efforts. When the choral hydrate was discontinued, the latter group continued to show improvement, while the former group got worse again. This seems to have important implications as to the nature of sleep disturbances following withdrawal of hypnotics, and on the role of the patient's understanding of the therapeutic process. The latter issue is a major concern in the next type of therapy to be discussed.

Behavioral Self-Management

The self-management approach of Coates and Thoresen (1977) emphasizes the need to acquire not only specific procedures such as progressive relaxation but also skills in assessing and solving problems related to insomnia. They point out that many behavioral techniques are administered in a manner similar to that used for a medication, i.e., it is expected that the method will be effective without the patient's being aware of the mechanism of action. Central to behavioral self-management is the concept that the patient is most effectively treated by learning skills which help him work out his own difficulties and by developing a belief that he is capable of using them effectively (Thoresen et al., in press). This sensation of mastery is important in countering what they consider to be an important complicating factor in insomnia—the patient's feeling of importance in dealing with the problem. As an example of a multifaceted treatment approach, they suggest that for one patient it may be insufficient to perform relaxation procedures at bedtime; this might be effective only after he also learns to manage his professional work time more efficiently in order to decrease daytime stress and the need to do anxiety-provoking work in the evening. The behavioral self-management approach has been reported to have been useful in six out of seven published cases, primarily of sleep-maintenance insomnia (including two adolescents), with favorable follow-up data after 6–36 months (Kirmil-Gray, Coates, Thoresen, Rosekind, & Price, 1978; Thoresen, Coates, Kirmil-Gray, & Rosekind, 1978).

SUMMARY AND CONCLUSIONS

Nonpharmacologic approaches to insomnia include office counseling, psychotherapy, and behavioral therapies. Office counseling is believed by many physicians to be of value. In addition to imparting information about conditions associated with insomnia and about "sleep hygiene," it is a useful vehicle for establishing a good physician–patient relationship. Psychotherapy has been advocated as a major form of treatment, although data on the efficacy for insomnia of this very time-consuming and expensive approach are not yet available.

A variety of behavioral techniques have been employed in efforts to improve sleep. Many of them are based on the hypothesis that insomniacs have difficulty falling asleep because of excessive autonomic stimulation, an idea which has not fared well in a variety of studies since it was propounded. A large group of behavioral approaches shares the common quality of attempting to enhance relaxation at bedtime by such methods as EMG biofeedback, progressive relaxation, and autogenic training. The data so far imply that these methods are of relatively little benefit to insomniacs as a whole, although the possibility exists that there is more improvement with biofeedback techniques which are individualized for the *type* of disturbance. Other treatments are derived from conditioning theories and include systematic desensitization and classical conditioning. The former has shown some benefits in a small group of uncontrolled studies, and in controlled conditions showed no more improvement than treatment with progressive relaxation alone. The latter has shown promise in individual case reports but as yet has not been tested in a controlled study. The stimulus–control approach, which attempts to eliminate behaviors incompatible with sleep from the bedroom environment, has been helpful in several studies. In one form of attribution therapy, subjects are encouraged to attribute their disturbed sleep to external, emotionally neutral sources; studies of effectiveness are contradictory, and it is doubtful whether this approach is very effective. An attempt to improve insomnia by encouraging the subject to attribute to himself the ability to fall asleep easily seemed promising and worthy of further exploration. The attribution therapies are interesting in that many deal with the patient's attitudes and expectations about hypnotics and the effect these may have on the efficacy of treatment. The behavioral self-management approach of Thoresen *et al.* (in press) emphasizes the need for the patient to acquire not only specific techniques such as progressive relaxation, but also the ability to assess and solve problems which may contribute to insomnia. It emphasizes the benefit of developing a sense of mastery, in order to counteract a feeling of impotence in dealing with the insomnia. Intensively examined cases have been encouraging, and this method seems well worthy of further investigation.

One difficulty in assessing the studies of behavioral therapists is that most of them have employed vaguely described groups of insomniacs, or "poor sleepers" who do not consider themselves to have a sleep disturbance. With the exception of the behavioral self-management group, there have been few efforts to separate out patients with sleep apnea, nocturnal myoclonus, or other conditions which are unlikely to be helped by behavioral therapies and hence might obscure possible benefits to other insomniac patients. When studies which look at subgroups of insomniacs are performed, it may be found that some forms of behavioral therapy will be useful for some patients.

CHAPTER 12

Conclusion: Implications for Medical Practice

SUMMARY

We are beginning to have some understanding of the phenomenology of sleep, but its function remains elusive. It may be studied in terms of the EEG sleep measures, but their relationship to the subjective qualities of sleep—e.g., loss of consciousness, a sense of restoration—are not entirely clear. Something about this experience of sleeping has gone amiss in the perhaps one-third of Americans who complain of sleeplessness or lack of refreshment. Studies of large numbers of these insomniacs show that although as a group they sleep less and take longer to go to sleep than noncomplaining individuals, the EEG measures of the two groups overlap substantially. This seems to indicate that factors other than a decrease in the total amount of EEG sleep are involved in the genesis of the uncomfortable experience of insomnia. Among these may be a dissociation of the usual relationship of the sensation of arousal to EEG-defined waking, disorders of the circadian rhythm of sleep, and disruptions of the nonREM/REM cycle by multiple brief awakenings. It is also becoming clear that insomniacs are a heterogeneous group, many of whom have specific disturbances such as sleep apnea, nocturnal myoclonus, and depressive illness.

The response of many persons—perhaps 5–15% of the population—to insomnia is to take prescription hypnotics at least occasionally, and 1–3% take them very frequently. An additional 6% or so, perhaps a different group from those who take prescription hypnotics, purchase over-the-counter sleep aids. Given this large rate of consumption, it behooves us to learn as much as possible about the characteristics of these agents, their benefits and possible hazards.

The pharmacology of the hypnotics is very diverse. They include a number of different chemical classes which vary in many qualities including the ease of absorption, biological half-life, route of excretion, presence of psychoactive metabolites, and other factors. One consequence of this diversity is that each drug has its own particular set of advantages and disadvantages. Thus no single hypnotic is generally "better," and in various clinical situations different hypnotics may be more advantageous (or at least less harmful).

The meaningfulness of evaluations of efficacy of hypnotics is limited by our very incomplete understanding of the nature of insomnia. It is not clear what the appropriate measures should be, and each of the commonly used approaches—the sleep EEG, patient reports, and nursing observations—have very clear limitations. In short-term use, virtually all prescription hypnotics have been reported to be more beneficial than placebo in some combination of these measures. Studies of longest duration in insomniacs have suggested that flurazepam increases total sleep for at least 28 days, but even this is shorter than the duration of the average hypnotic prescription. Studies in normal volunteers have also reported increased total sleep with chloral hydrate for 28 days and with nitrazepam for over 10 weeks. Whether this translates into effectiveness for insomniacs is not known. There are virtually no available studies of efficacy during intermittent usage, which may well be the most common way these agents are taken in practice. This problem is compounded by the almost complete lack of longitudinal data on the natural course of patients with various types of insomnia.

It is not at all clear which patients should be given hypnotics. Most investigators agree that hypnotics have limited usefulness when insomnia is accompanied by an associated disorder such as nocturnal myoclonus or phase lag syndrome. It has been argued that among the remaining patients with "primary" insomnia, only those with objective EEG evidence of disturbed sleep should be given hypnotics; others believe that the subjective experience of insomnia sufficiently justifies the use of hypnotics. The former argument appeals to scientific rigor, but at present limits the prescribing of hypnotics to a minority of patients. Another difficulty is that our ability to define objective disturbances of sleep is changing constantly. As but one example, the use of multivariate analysis may rapidly increase the percentage of patients who can be objectively identified as insomniacs. The second problem is that many drugs, including tranquilizers, antidepressants, and analgesics, are often given on the basis of the patient's reports of his subjective feelings and behavior; it is not clear that an electronic measure of disturbed physiology is needed before a medication is given. These are, however, nothing but speculations, best resolved by the outcome of careful follow-up studies, which are waiting to be performed.

Although systematic hypnotic efficacy studies are generally incomplete and suggest limited usefulness of hypnotics, these agents are of course very widely prescribed and many practitioners claim to see benefits which exceed those documented by investigators. Similarly, several polls of large populations of users report that a large proportion—80% in one study—believe that their prescription hypnotics help them substantially. The sources of this discrepancy are not clear. It is possible that the patients are experiencing a placebo effect, or that sleeping pills serve some beneficial function in the physician's relationship to a patient seeking help, or that hypnotics produce some other effect (such as euphoria or tranquilization) which is unrelated to sleep but which places them in high demand. Alternatively, it may be that both patients and many physicians are recognizing some clinical benefit which is not picked up in systematic studies—in short, investigators might not be measuring the right things. There is also a possibility that although benefit to *groups* of patients are very modest in systematic studies, some individual patients are helped greatly.

In contrast to our very tentative knowledge about the efficacy of hypnotics, evidence is accumulating rapidly about the many hazards of widespread hypnotic use. The importance of this problem was emphasized by a prospective population study now several years old which suggested that persons with no history of medical illness but who used hypnotics often were 1.5 times more likely to die in the next 6 years than those who never used such drugs. The negative aspects of hypnotic use which have received the most attention are toxicity in acute overdose and drug addiction. Although these are very real problems, it is essential not to lose sight of others which are often less dramatic but still very important. These include interactions with other drugs (including ethanol), daytime residual effects, and enhanced toxicity in the elderly.

The interaction of hypnotics with ethanol must be carefully assessed, as they are frequently taken together in both routine use and overdose. There is a growing literature on the relation of ethanol–hypnotic interactions on driving skills. Although the interpretation of these studies is difficult, the very least that can be said is that many drivers who are arrested or are involved in accidents have been taking both ethanol and a hypnotic or anxiolytic, and it behooves us to understand the effects of such combinations. Studies of ethanol–hypnotic interactions indicate that performance may be affected variably, depending on which measure is used, dose, duration of administration, and other factors. The potential for adverse interactions also varies for different drugs in the same chemical class. Diazepam, for instance, seems more clearly to interact with ethanol than do some other benzodiazepines such as chlordiazepoxide or oxazepam. There is relatively little work on the combination of ethanol with flurazepam, although this drug accounts for over half of all hypnotic prescriptions.

Since the half-lives of many hypnotics are substantially longer than 8 hr, one consequence of taking hypnotics is that a patient may have substantial amounts of active drug in his body during the daytime. Hypnotics may alter the waking EEG up to 18 hr after administration; although the clinical significance is uncertain, this at least demonstrates that these agents continue to have physiological effects well into the next day after bedtime use. Tests of psychomotor function show a variety of deficits at least 16–19 hr after a single dose, and over the entire day during chronic administration. Although the relation of such tests to practical skills such as driving is not entirely clear, these results certainly raise the possibility that persons who take hypnotics may have decreased performance in practical daytime chores. Perhaps most worrisome is the finding that persons with drug-induced performance deficits may be subjectively unaware of their impairment.

The elderly may be particularly at risk for deleterious residual effects or toxic reactions to hypnotics. This may stem from increased nervous system sensitivity, as well as altered absorption, distribution, and excretion of drugs. Decreased clearance and/or increased volume of distribution of many hypnotics may lead to prolonged plasma half-lives of these agents in the elderly. Any clinical difficulties associated with this would seem likely to be magnified with the traditional benzodiazepines such as flurazepam, which even in young adults have both psychoactive metabolites and substantially longer half-lives than most other hypnotics. Empirically, the incidence of toxic reactions to flurazepam does increase with age, and in one study was a problem in one-fourth of nursing home patients receiving it. Disinhibition reactions in the elderly resulting in restlessness and aggression have long been associated with the barbiturates but may occur in all classes of hypnotics. All of these problems are compounded by the disproportionately high rate of use of hypnotics by the elderly. In contrast, hypnotics are tested most extensively in young adults. Thus we tend to test hypnotics in one generation and then administer them to another.

All of the hazards of hypnotic use would seem to be enhanced by the tendency for many persons—perhaps 15–20% of those started on hypnotics—to continue to take them for prolonged periods. A large number of these chronic users—over 20% in one study—were started on these agents while hospitalized for medical, surgical, or psychiatric disorders. There is also some evidence that prolonged usage may develop in patients who seem medically and psychologically healthy, but are given hypnotics during a period of stress. Tentative data suggest that patients started on those hypnotics which are not generally considered to have substantial abuse potential, such as nitrazepam, may be as likely to desire long-term use as those started on amobarbital. The factors which contribute to such long-term use are not clear, and need to be studied. As but one example, it is uncertain to what degree disturbed sleep from withdrawal of clinical doses contributes to a desire to continue medication, nor is it documented how frequently such sleep disturbance occurs.

Alternative approaches to the use of prescription hypnotics include OTC hypnotics and nonpharmacologic treatments for insomnia. The OTC hypnotics are used perhaps even more widely than their prescription counterparts. The few efficacy studies which are available show mixed results, and studies of what until recently have been the two major ingredients have indicated a carcinogenic risk from one (methapyrilene) and a tendency for toxic anticholinergic effects from the other (scopolamine aminoxide). Developments in the large and lucrative market for OTC hypnotics should be carefully followed.

The most common nonpharmacologic approaches to insomnia are the traditional forms of psychotherapy and behavior modification techniques. Although the experience of many psychotherapists leads them to believe in the efficacy of their approach, there are no available systematic studies demonstrating substantial benefits to insomniacs. Many of the behavioral approaches to treating insomnia are based on the questionable hypothesis that excessive autonomic stimulation is important in keeping patients from sleeping. Systematic studies of techniques to enhance relaxation such as EMG biofeedback, autogenic training, and progressive relaxation suggest that they are of little benefit to groups of insomniacs. Two techniques which may have the most promise are stimulus control and behavioral self-management, although they first need to pass the test of controlled trials. One of the difficulties in this area has been that most studies were done on groups of insomniacs who have not been subjected to careful diagnosis of associated conditions (e.g., sleep apnea) unlikely to be helped by these techniques. Thus it may be that some nonpharmacologic methods are beneficial to selected patients, but that these benefits are obscured in studies of heterogeneous groups of insomniacs.

We are faced, then, with large numbers of Americans seeking help for insomnia, while the therapeutic armamentarium, although varied and widely used, has little scientific support. Our meager understanding of insomnia and of the possible benefits of available hypnotics cannot justify a conclusive set of recommendations for the use of hypnotics at this time. It might be well, however, to end by briefly summarizing a practical approach to the insomniac patient and some tentative conclusions on the use of hypnotics.

APPROACH TO THE INSOMNIAC PATIENT

Evaluation

As in any other area of medicine, a careful history is essential. The goals should be to:

1. *Characterize the complaint.* Is the main problem difficulty falling asleep, awakenings during the night, early-morning arousal, or some combination of these? Does the patient feel refreshed in the morning? How long has this problem gone on? Does it represent a clear change in the patient's usual habits?

2. *Get a sense of his usual habits.* When does he usually go to sleep and get up? Does he take daytime naps? Are his sleep hours relatively fixed or variable?

3. *Determine general medical health.* Are there illnesses present which might produce discomfort associated with disturbed sleep? Arthritis, for instance, may produce pain which keeps the patient awake. Diabetes mellitus or treatment with diuretics may result in awakenings to urinate at night. Patients with congestive heart failure may have dyspnea when supine. In view of the tentative evidence linking benzodiazepines and barbiturates with birth defects and brain tumors, one should also determine if the patient is pregnant.

4. *Determine if he is taking other medicines.* Is his insomnia related to use of multiple doses of hypnotics each night? Is he taking anxiolytics or other drugs which might potentiate the effects of hypnotics? Is he on anticoagulants or other drugs whose metabolism or protein binding might be affected by hypnotics? Does he regularly take ethanol or drugs of abuse?

5. *Examine the possibility of depressive illness or other psychiatric disorders.* This is particularly vital because depression is so common (affecting perhaps 5–9% of men and women sometime during their lives) and because half of patients with depressive illness go to physicians complaining primarily of some "somatic" symptom such as insomnia, rather than

depressed mood. One should inquire whether the patient has lost interest in activities he used to enjoy, and whether he has feelings of hoplessness or suicidal thoughts. Both clinical experience and some EEG data (e.g., Gillin et al., 1979) indicate that early-morning awakenings are more commonly associated with the sleep disturbance of depression than with other forms of insomnia.

6. *Determine if there are other associated conditions, in which treatment with hypnotics is likely to be ineffective (e.g., nocturnal myoclonus) or harmful (e.g., sleep apnea), or for which there are nonpharmacological approaches (e.g., phase lag syndrome).* Does the patient snore a great deal? (It is often helpful to have a patient bring in a tape recording made during sleep and to play it in the background during the interview.) Does he kick his bed partner or tear up the bedclothes at night? (On questions such as these, an interview with the bed partner is obviously very useful.) Does he cough and gag during sleep (perhaps indicating gastroesophageal problems)?

7. *Determine whether he has an increased risk of harm from taking hypnotics.* Persons who fall into this category include those who have liver or renal disease, are elderly, are depressed (because of increased potential for suicide), are taking other medications which might adversely interact with hypnotics, have a history of drug abuse, or have occupations (e.g., flying) in which small errors in judgment or coordination might have life-threatening consequences.

The Decision Whether to Give Hypnotics

When an associated condition is found, the approach should be to give specific treatment rather than reflexively attempting relief with hypnotics. For a depressed patient with sleep disturbance, the correct therapeutic response is to give antidepressants such as the tricyclics or monoamine oxidase inhibitors; it is not at all clear that hypnotics add anything useful to this regimen. Similarly, when insomnia seems related to the discomfort of a medical illness (e.g., arthritis), the appropriate response is to adjust medications more relevant to the illness (in this case, perhaps antiinflammatory agents and analgesics) rather than routinely prescribing a hypnotic. As another example, patients on diuretics can sometimes be given their medicine earlier in the day to reduce arousals from a full bladder.

The decision remains, then, of how to treat those patients in whom various associated disorders have been ruled out. At this time one can only make judgments in the absence of adequate data. The following tentative thoughts, which have helped guide this author, are divided according to whether the problem is acute or more long lasting.

Acute or Intermittent Insomnia

The available data lend some support to giving hypnotics for brief periods to persons whose sleep is temporarily disturbed by an acute stress (e.g., bereavement or hospitalization). On the other hand, there is some evidence that prescribing to individuals who are in the midst of a disturbing situation or who are entering the hospital often leads to prolonged use; moreover, hospitalized patients may be at particular risk for undesirable drug interactions. Another problem is posed by the patient with an occasional night of poor sleep, who desires hypnotics on an "as needed" basis. There are virtually no systematic data on efficacy in this situation, but the preponderance of ancedotal data suggests that they might be used in this manner with patients who are well known to the physician.

Chronic Insomnia

The crucial issue here is whether the patient is already on hypnotics. If he is not taking them, it seems unwise to prescribe medication which has never been shown to be of help over an extended period of time. This is the patient for whom one intuitively suspects that counseling, discussions of "sleep hygiene" (e.g., regularizing his time of going to bed, etc.), and nonpharmacologic behavioral approaches should be tried. A second issue is raised by a group about whom one often hears, but who are poorly documented—those patients, often elderly, who have already been receiving recommended doses for many years and who are content with their sleep. Here there are no clear answers, but one could argue that it is reasonable to continue such medication, with eternal vigilance to prevent escalating dosages. Finally, there are those patients with chronic insomnia taking massive doses of hypnotics, as discussed in Chapter 8. These might be particularly good candidates for referral to a sleep disorder center. The general treatment, as outlined before, is gradual withdrawal of medication.

When Hypnotics Are Prescribed

If one chooses to give a hypnotic, the efficacy data are so ambiguous that the choice of a particular drug is best made by assessing their relative risks. The preferable agent may vary with the situation. For instance, a drug which is dangerous in acute overdose but has other advantages may reasonably be used in the controlled setting of a hospital. Similarly, a hypnotic with a particularly long half-life but relatively low toxicity in acute overdose may be useful in a young adult but perhaps less appropriate in an elderly patient.

When hypnotics are prescribed, the patient needs to be given realistic (and limited) expectations of benefit. It should be emphasized that these drugs have at best a short-term usefulness. The problem of tolerance should be discussed, and it should be made clear that increasing the dosage, although tempting, is a perilous path. In language designed to inform rather than to frighten, one should tell the patient about the hazards of overdose, the interaction with ethanol and other drugs, and the possibility of effects on daytime functioning.

Finally, it is important to prescribe hypnotics in small quantities, without automatic refills. One useful approach is to list specific goals (e.g., to decrease difficulty falling asleep) in the medical record; subsequent notes can be used to evaluate whether the hypnotic is helping achieve them. The patient should be carefully monitored for side effects, as well as unilateral increases in dosage (which are often associated with later dependence). If one has first conditioned the patient to the notion that hypnotics will only be used briefly, and that they are not a panacea, later encouragement to discontinue their use will be much easier.

References

Abe, K., and Shimakawa, M. Genetic-constitutional factor and childhood insomnia. *Psychiat. Neurol. 152:*363–369, 1966.

Abelson, H. I., Fishburne, P. M., and Cisin, I. *National survey on drug abuse: 1977*, vol. 1. National Institute on Drug Abuse, DHEW publication (ADM) 78–618, 1977, p. 105.

Adam, K., Adamson, L., Březinová, V., Hunter, W. M., and Oswald, I. Nitrazepam: Lastingly effective but trouble on withdrawal. *Br. Med. J.* 1:1558–1560, 1976.

Adamson, J., and Burdick, J. A. Sleep of dry alcoholics. *Arch. Gen. Psychiatry 28:*146–149, 1973.

Agnew, H. W., and Webb, W. B. Sleep latencies in human subjects: Age, prior wakefulness, and reliability. *Psychonomic Science 24:*253–254, 1971.

Agnew, H. W., Webb, W. B., and Williams, R. L. The effects of stage four sleep deprivation. *Electroencephalogr. Clin. Neurophysiol. 27:*68–70, 1964.

Allen, R. P., Wagman, A., Faillace, L. A., and McIntosh, M. Electroencepholographic (EEG) sleep recovery following prolonged alcohol intoxication in alcoholics. *J. Nerv. Ment. Dis. 153:*424–433, 1971.

Allgulander, C. Dependence on sedative and hypnotic drugs—a comparative clinical and social study. *Acta Psychiatr. Scand. Suppl. 270:*1–102, 1978.

Allgulander, C., and Borg, S. Case report: A delirious abstinence syndrome associated with clorazepate "Tranxilen." *Br. J. Addict.*, in press.

Allnutt, M. F., and O'Connor, P. J. Comparison of the electrocencephalographic, behavioral and subjective correlates of natural and drug-induced sleep at atypical hours. *Aerosp. Med. 42:*1006–1010, 1971.

Alvan, G., Lindgren, J. E., Bogentoft, C., and Ericsson, O. Plasma kinetics of methaqualone in man after single oral doses. *Eur. J. Clin. Pharmacol. 6:*187–190, 1973.

Alvan, G., Ericsson, O., Levander, S., and Lindgren, J. Plasma concentrations and effects of methaqualone after single and multiple oral doses in man. *Eur. J. Clin. Pharmacol. 7:*449–454, 1974.

Ananth, J. V., Bonheim, L. A., Klinger, A., and Ban, T. A. Diazepam in the treatment of insomnia in psychiatric patients. *Curr. Ther. Res. Clin. Exp. 15:*217–222, 1973.

Andersen, T., and Lingjaerde, O. Nitrazepam (Mogodan) as a sleep inducing agent. *Br. J. Psychiatr. 115:*1393–1397, 1969.

187

Arieff, A. I., and Friedman, E. A. Coma following non-narcotic drug overdose: Management of 208 adult patients. *Am. J. Med. Sci. 266*:405–426, 1973.

Asbell, N. Clinical evaluation of a new nonbarbiturate sedative hypnotic, 2-methyl-3-o-tolyl-4-quinazolone: Double-blind study. *J. Am. Geriatr. Soc. 10*:1032–1037, 1962.

Ascione, F. J. Evaluating drug interactions: Benzodiazepines with alcohol. *Drug Therapy 1*:58–71, 1978.

Aserinsky, E., and Kleitman, N. Regularly occurring periods of eye motility, and concomitant phenomena during sleep. *Science 118*:273–274, 1953.

Auwers, K., and von Meyenburg, F. Ueber eine neue Synthese von Derivaten des Isin-dazoles. *Ber. Dtsch. Chem. Ges. 24*:2370–2388, 1891.

Aviado, D. M. *Pharmacologic Principles of Medical Practice.* Williams and Wilkins, Baltimore, 1972, pp. 56–90.

Baekeland, F. Pentobarbital and dertroaniphetamine sulphate: Effects on sleep cycle in man. *Psychopharmacologia 11*:388–396, 1967.

Baile, W. F., DePaulo, J. R., Jr., and Schmidt, C. W., Jr. Emergency room management of organic brain syndromes caused by over-the-counter hypnotics. *Md. State Med. J. 26*:61–63, 1977.

Balasubramaniam, K., Lucas, S. B., Mawer, G. E., and Simons, P. J. The kinetics of amylobarbitone metabolism in healthy men and women. *Br. J. Pharmacol. 39*:564–572, 1970.

Balasubramaniam, K., Mawer, G. E., Pohl, J. E. F., and Simons, P. J. G. Impairment of cognitive functions associated with hydroxyamylobarbitone accumulation in patients with renal insufficiency. *Br. J. Pharmacol. 45*:360–367, 1972.

Ballinger, B. R., Presly, A., Reid, A. H., and Stevenson, I. H. The effects of hypnotics on imipramine treatment. *Psychopharmacologia 39*:267–274, 1974.

Ballinger, C. B. Subjective sleep disturbance at the menopause. *J. Psychosom. Res. 20*(5):509–513, 1976.

Balter, M. B., and Bauer, M. Patterns of prescribing and use of hypnotic drugs in the United States, *in Sleep Disturbance and Hypnotic Drug Dependence*, Clift, A. D. (ed.), Excerpta Medica, Amsterdam, 1975, pp. 261–293.

Ban, T. A., and McGinnis, K. Comparative clinical study of two hypnotic drugs. *Can. Med. Assoc. J. 87*:816–817, 1962.

Bancroft, J. H., Skrimshire, A. M., Reynolds, F., Simkin, S., and Smith, J. Self-poisoning and self-injury in the Oxford area: Epidemiological aspects 1969–1973. *Brit. J. Prev. and Soc. Med. 29*:170–177, 1975.

Bartholini, G., Keller, H., Pieri, L., and Pletscher, A. The effect of diazepam on the turnover of cerebral dopamine, *in The Benzodiazepines*, Garattini, S., Mussini, E., and Pandall, L. O. (eds.), Rowen Press, New York, 1973, pp. 235–240.

Battegay, R. Sucht nach Abusus von Doriden. *Praxis 46*:991–992, 1957.

Bayne, W. F., Tao, F. T., and Crisologo, N. Submicrogram assay for scopolamine in plasma and urine. *J. Pharm. Sci. 64*:288–291, 1975.

Beilin, P. E. An attempt to organize medical treatment by conditioned reflex sleep in the Makarov Hospital. *Klin. Med. (Vienna) 9*:50–58, 1952.

Bender, A. D. Pharmacodynamic principles of drug therapy in the aged. *J. Am. Geriatr. Soc. 22*:296–303, 1974.

Berger, H. Das Electroencephalogram des Menschen. *Arch. Psychiatr. Nervenkr. 87*:527–570, 1929.

Berger, P. A., and Tinklenberg, J. R. Treatment of abusers of alcohol and other addictive drugs, *in Psycho-Pharmacology: From Theory to Practice*, Barchos, J. D., Berger, P. A., Ciaranello, R. D., and Elliott, G. R. (eds.), Oxford University Press, New York, 1977, pp. 355–385.

Berger, R. S. Tonus of extrinsic laryngeal muscles during sleep and dreaming. *Science* 134:840, 1961.

Bernstine, J. B., Meyer, A. E., and Bernstine, R. L. Maternal blood and breast milk estimation following adminstration of chloral hydrate during puerperium. *J. Obstet. Gynaecol. Br. Emp.* 63:228–231, 1956.

Billiard, M., Besset, A., and Passouant, P. Screening a population of insomniacs. *Sleep Res.* 5:159, 1976.

Billiard, M., Besset, A., Passouant, P. Strategy for treatment of chronic insomnia. *Sleep Res.* 7:209, 1978.

Bixler, E. O., Kales, A., Tan, T. L., and Kales, J. D. The effects of hypnotic drugs on performance. *Curr. Ther. Res. Clin. Exp.* 15:13–24, 1973.

Bixler, E., Saldatos, C., Kales, A., and Russek, E. Prevalence of sleep apnea in chronic insomniacs. *Sleep Res.* 5:161, 1976.

Bixler, E. O., Kales, A., Soldatos, C. R., Scharf, M. B., and Kales, J. D. Effectiveness of temazepam with short-, intermediate-, and long-term use: Sleep laboratory evaluation. *J. Clin. Pharmacol.* 18:110–118, 1978.

Bixler, E. O., Soldatos, C. R., Scarone, S., Martin, E. D., Kales, A., and Charney, D. S. Similarities of nocturnal myoclonic activity in insomniac patients and normal subjects. *Sleep Res.* 7:213, 1978.

Blacow, N. W. *Martindale: The extra pharmacopoeia,* 26th ed. The Pharmaceutical Press, London, 1972, pp. 890–930.

Blake, W. Some effects of pentobarbital anaesthesia on renal hemodynamics, water and electrolyte excretion in the dog. *Am. J. Physiol.* 191:393–398, 1957.

Bloomfield, S. S., Tetreault, L., Lafreniere, B., and Bordeleau, J. M. A method for the evaluation of hypnotic agents in man. The comparative hypnotic effects of secobarbital, methaqualone and placebo in normal subjects and in psychiatric patients. *J. Pharmacol. Exp. Therapeutics* 156(2):375–382, 1967.

Bo, O., Haffner, J. F. W., Langard, O., Trumpy, J. H., Bredesen, J. E., and Lunde, P. K. M. Ethanol and diazepam as causative factors in traffic accidents, in *Proceedings,* Sixth International Conference on Alcohol and Traffic, Israelstam, S., and Langer, E. (eds.), Toronto, 1976.

Bogan, J., and Smith, H. The relation between primidone and phenobarbitone blood levels. *J. Pharm. Pharmacol.* 20:64–67, 1968.

Bond, A. J., and Lader, M. H. Residual effects of hypnotics. *Psychopharmacologia* 25:117–132, 1972.

Bond, A. J., and Lader, M. H. The residual effects of flurazepam. *Psychopharmacologia* 32:223–235, 1973.

Bond, A. J., and Lader, M. H. Residual effects of flunitrazepam. *Br. J. Clin. Pharmacol.* 2:143–150, 1975.

Bootzin, R. R. Stimulus control treatment for insomnia. *Proceedings, Am. Psychol. Assoc.* 395–396, Honolulu, Hawaii, 1972.

Bootzin, R. R. Stimulus control of insomnia. Paper presented at the meeting of the Am. Psychol. Assoc., Montreal, 1973.

Bootzin, R. R. Stimulus control treatment of insomnia. Paper presented at the meeting of the Am. Psychol. Assoc., Chicago, 1974.

Bootzin, R. R. Effects of self-control procedures for insomnia, *in Behavioral Self-Management,* Stuart, R. B. (ed.). Brunner/Mazel, New York, 1977, pp. 176–195.

Bootzin, R. R., Herman, C. P., and Nicassio, P. The power of suggestion: Another examination of misattribution and insomnia. *J. Pers. Soc. Psychol.* 34:673–679, 1976.

Borkovec, T. C., and Fowles, D. C. Controlled investigation of the effects of progressive and hypnotic relaxation on insomnia. *J. Abnorm. Psychol.* 82:153–158, 1973.

Borkovec, T. C., Steinmark, S., and Nau, S. Relaxation training and single-item desensitization in the group treatment of insomnia. *J. Behav. Ther. Exp. Psychiatry* 4:401–403, 1973.

Borland, R. G., and Nicholson, A. N. Comparison of the residual effects of two benzodiazepines (nitrazepam and flurazepam hydrochloride) and pentobarbitone sodium on human performance. *Br. J. Clin. Pharmacol.* 2:9–17, 1975.

Boston Collaborative Drug Surveillance Program. A clinical evaluation of flurazepam. *J. Clin. Pharmacol.*, May–June 1972, pp. 217–220.

Boston Collaborative Drug Surveillance Program. Clinical depression of the central nervous system due to diazepam and chlordiazepoxide in relation to cigarette smoking and age. *N. Engl. J. Med.* 288(6):277–280, 1973.

Brazier, M. A. B. *The Electrical Activity of the Nervous System.* Pitman Medical, Great Britain, pp. 227–239.

Breckenridge, A., and Orme, M. Clinical implications of enzyme induction. *Ann. N.Y. Acad. Sci.* 179:421–431, 1971.

Breimer, D. D. Pharmacokinetics and biopharmaceutical aspects of hypnotic drug therapy, in *Clinical Pharmacy and Clinical Pharmacology,* Gouveia, W. A., Tognoni, G., and Van der Kleijn, E. (eds.), New York: North Holland, 1976a, pp. 17–42.

Breimer, D. D. Pharmacokinetics of methohexitone following intravenous infusion in humans. *Br. J. Anaesth.* 48:643–649, 1976b.

Breimer, D. D. Clinical pharmacokinetics of hypnotics. *Clin. Pharmacokinet.* 2:93–109, 1977.

Breimer, D. D., and DeBoer, A. G. Pharmacokinetics and relative bioavailability of heptabarbital and heptabarbital sodium in man after oral administration. *Eur. J. Clin. Pharmacol.* 9:169–178, 1975.

Breimer, D. D., and DeBoer, A. G. Pharmacokinetics and relative bioavailability of vinylbital in man after oral and rectal administration. *Arzneim. Forsch.* 26:448–454, 1976.

Breimer, D. D., and Van Rossum, J. M. Pharmacokinetics of (+) and (−) and (±) hexobarbitone in man after oral administration. *J. Pharm. Pharmacol.* 25:762–764, 1973.

Breimer, D. D., and Winten, M. A. C. M. Pharmacokinetics and relative bioavailability of cyclobarbital calcium in man after oral administration. *Eur. J. Clin. Pharmacol.* 9:443–450, 1976.

Breimer, D. D., Ketelaars, H. C. J., and Van Rossum, J. M. The determination of chloral hydrate, trichloroethanol and trichoroacetic acid in blood and urine, employing deadspace analysis. *J. Chromatogr.* 88:55–63, 1974.

Breimer, D. D., Honhoff, C., Zilly, W., Richter, E., and Van Rossum, J. M. Pharmacokinetics of hexobarbital in man after intravenous infusion. *J. Pharmacokinet. Biopharm.* 3:1–11, 1975.

Breimer, D. D., Zilly, W., and Richter, E. Pharmacokinetics of hexobarbital in acute hepatitis and after apparent recovery. *Clin. Pharmacol. Ther.* 18:443–440, 1975.

Bridges-Webb, C. Attempted suicide by drug overdose in a country town. *Med. J. Australia* 2:782–783, 1973.

Brodie, B. B. Distribution and fate of drugs: Therapeutic implications, in *Absorption and Distribution of Drugs,* Binns, T. B. (ed.). Livingstone, Edinburgh, 1964, pp. 199–200.

Broughton, R. Neurochemical, neuroendocrine and biorythmic aspects of sleep in man: Relationship to clinical pathological disorders. *Adv. Behav. Biol.* 10:359–397, 1973.

Brouschek, R., and Feuerlein, M. Valamin als suchtmittel. *Nervenarzt* 27:115–117, 1956.

Brown, W. T. A comparative study of three hypnotics: Methyprylon, glutethimide, and chloral hydrate. *Can. Med. Assoc. J.* 102:510–511, 1970.

Brownman, C. P., Gordon, G. C., Tepas, D. I., and Walsh, J. K. Reported sleep and drug habits of workers: A preliminary report. *Sleep Res.* 6:111, 1977.

Bryan, G. T. The role of urinary tryptophan metabolites in the etiology of bladder cancer. *J. Clin. Nutr.* 24:841–847, 1971.

Budzynski, T. H. Biofeedback procedures in the clinic. *Semin. Psychiatry* 5:537–547, 1973.

Budzynski, T. H., Stoyva, J., and Adler, C. Feedback-induced relaxation: Application to tension headache. *J. Behav. Ther. Exp. Psychiatry* 1:205–211, 1970.

Burke, A. W. Attempted suicide in Trinidad and Tobago. *West Indian Med. J.* 23:250–255, 1974.

Cahn, C. H. Intoxication to ethclorvynol (Placidyl). *Can. Med. Assoc. J.* 81:733–734, 1959.

Calloway, N. O., and Merrill, R. S. The aging adult liver. I. Bromsulphalein and bilirubin clearances. *J. Am. Geriatr. Soc.* 13:594, 1965.

Carmichael, F. J., and Israel, Y. Effect of ethanol on neurotransmitter release by rat brain cortical slices. *J. Pharmacol. Exp. Ther.* 193:824–834, 1975.

Carskadon, M. A., Dement, W. C., Mitler, M. M., Guilleminault, C., Zarcone, V. P., and Spiegel, R. Self-reports versus sleep laboratory findings in 122 drug-free subjects with complaints of chronic insomnia. *Am. J. Psychiatry* 133:1382–1383, 1476, 1976.

Caton, R. Description of a new form of recording apparatus for the use of practical physiology classes. *J. Anat. Physiol.* 22:103–106, 1887.

Chia, B. H., and Tsoi, W. F. A statistical study of attempted suicides in Singapore. *Singapore Med. J.* 15:253–256, 1974.

Chung, H., and Brown, D. R. Alcohol–hexobarbital interaction in rats under acute stress. *Life Sci.* 18:123–128, 1976.

Church, M. W., and Johnson, L. C. Mood and performance of poor sleepers during repeated use of flurazepam. *Psychopharmacol.* 61:309–316, 1979.

Clark, D. L., and Rosner, B. S. Neurophysiologic effects of general anaesthetics. I. The electroencephalogram and sensory evoked responses in man. *Anaesthesiology* 38:564–582, 1973.

Clemes, S., and Dement, W. The effect of REM sleep deprivation on psychological functioning. *J. Nerv. Ment. Dis.* 144:485–491, 1967.

Clemmesen, C., and Nilsson, E. Therapeutic trends in the treatment of barbiturate poisoning. *Clin. Pharmacol. Ther.* 2(2):220–229, 1961.

Clifford, J. M., Cookson, J. H., and Wickham, P. E. Absorption and clearance of secobarbital, hetabarbital, methaqualone and ethinamate. *Clin. Pharmacol. Ther.* 16:376–389, 1974.

Clift, A. D. A general practice study of dependence on some non-barbiturate hypnotic drugs, in *Sleep Disturbance and Hypnotic Drug Dependence*, Clift, A. D. (ed.), Excerpta Medica, New York, 1975a, pp. 97–105.

Clift, A. D. Sleep disturbance in general practice, in *Sleep Disturbance and Hypnotic Drug Dependence*, Clift, A. D. (ed.), Excerpta Medica, Armsterdam, 1975b, pp. 155–177.

Clift, A. D. Prediction of the dependence-prone patient: A general practice investigation, in *Sleep Disturbance and Hypnotic Drug Dependence*, Clift, A. D. (ed.), Excerpta Medica, Amsterdam, 1975c, pp. 107–153.

Coates, T. J., and Thoresen, C. E. *How to Sleep Better: A Drug Free Program for Overcoming Insomnia*. Prentice-Hall, Englewood Cliffs, N.J., 1977, pp. 1–324.

Cocchi, R., and Tornati, A. Psychic dependence: A different formulation of the problem with a view to the reorientation of therapy for chronic drug addiction. *Acta Psychiatr. Scand.* 56:337–346, 1977.

Coldwell, B. B., Wiberg, G. S., and Trenholm, H. L. Some effects of ethanol on the toxicity and distribution of barbiturates in rats. *Can J. Physiol. Pharmacol.* 48:254–264, 1970.

Conney, A. H., Davison, C., Gastel, R., and Burns, J. J. Adaptive increases in drug-metabolizing enzymes induced by phenobarbital and other drugs. *J. Pharmacol. Exp. Ther.* 130:1–8, 1960.

Conrad, R. D., and Kahn, M. W. An epidemiological study of suicide and attempted suicide among the Papago Indians. *Am. J. Psychiat.* 131:69–72, 1974.

Consolo, S., Garattini, S., and Ladinsky, H. Action of benzodiazepines on the cholinergic system. *Adv. Biochem. Psychopharmacol. 14*:63–80, 1975.

Cooper, J. R. *Sedative-hypnotic Drugs: Risks and Benefits*. National Institute on Drug Abuse, U.S. Department of Health, Education and Welfare, 1977, p. 69.

Costa, E., Guidotti, A., and Mao, C. C. Evidence for involvement of GABA in the action of benzodiazepines: Studies on rat cerebellum. *Adv. Biochem. Psychopharmacol. 14*:113–130, 1975.

Coursey, R. D., Buchsbaum, M., and Frankel, B. L. Personality measures and evoked responses in chronic insomniacs. *J. Abnorm. Psychol. 84*:239–249, 1975.

Craig, T. J., and Van Natta, P. A. Current medication use and symptoms of depression in a general population. *Am. J. Psychiatry 135*(9):1036–1039, 1978.

Crigler, J. F., and Gold, N. I. Effect of sodium phenobarbital on bilirubin metabolism in an infant with congenital nonhemolytic unconjugated hyperbilirubenemia and kernicterus. *J. Clin. Invest. 48*:42–55, 1969.

Crossland, J., and Slater, P. The effects of some drugs on the "free" and "bound" acetylcholine content of rat brain. *Br. J. Pharmacol. 33*:42, 1968.

Crowley, T. J., and Hydinger-Macdonald, M. Bedtime flurazepam and the human circadian rhythm of spontaneous motility. *Psychopharmacol. 62*:157–161, 1979.

Cucinell, S. A., Oddesky, L., Weiss, M., and Dayton, P. G. The effect of chloral hydrate on bishydroxycoumarin metabolism. *J. Am. Med. Assoc. 197*:366–368, 1966.

Curry, S. H., Riddall, D., Gordon, J. S., Simpson, P., Binns, T. B., Rondel, R. K., and McMartin, C. Disposition of glutethimide in man. *Clin. Pharmacol. Ther. 12*:849–857, 1971.

Czerwenka-Wenkstetten, H., Hofman, G., and Krypsin-Exner, K. Ein Fall von Valium-Entzugsdelir, *Wien. Med. Wochenschr. 47*:994–995, 1965.

Dalton, W. S., Martz, R., Rodda, B. E., Lemberger, L., and Forney, R. B. Influence of cannabidiol on secobarbital effects and plasma kinetics. *Clin. Pharmacol. Ther. 20*:695–700, 1976.

Davidson, G. L., Tsujimoto, R. N., and Glaros, A. G. Attribution and the maintence of behavior change in falling asleep. *J. Abnorm. Psychol. 82*:124–133, 1973.

Davies, C., and Levine, S. A controlled comparison of nitrazepam (Mogadon) with sodium amobarbitone as a sleep-inducing agent. *Br. J. Psychiatry 113*:1005–1008, 1967.

Dawborn, J. K., Turner, A., and Polkson, G. Ethchlorvynol as a sedative in patients with renal failure. *Med. J. Aust. 2*:702–704, 1972.

Dawson-Butterworth, K. The chemopsychotherapeutics of geriatric sedation. *J. Am. Geriatr. Soc. 18*(2):97–114, 1970.

DeGroot, G., Maes, A. A., and Van Heyst, A. N. P. The use of haemoperfusion in the elimination of absorbed drug mixtures in acute intoxication. *Neth. J. Med. 20*:142–148, 1977.

Dement, W. L. Experimental dream studies, in *Academy of Psychoanalysis: Science and Psychoanalysis*, Marserman, J. H. (ed.), Grune & Stratton, New York, 1964, pp. 129–184.

Dement, W. Recent studies on the biological role of REM sleep. *Am. J. Psychiatry 122*:404–408, 1965.

Dement, W. C. *Some Must Watch While Others Sleep*. Stanford, Calif., Stanford Alumni Association, 1973, pp. 5–8.

Dement, W., and Kleitman, N. Cyclic variations in EEG during sleep and their relation to eye movements, body motility and dreaming. *Electroencephalogr. Clin. Neurophysiol. 9*:673–690, 1957.

Dement, W. C., Mitler, M. M., and Henriksen, S. J. Sleep changes during chronic administration of parachlorophenylalanine. *Rev. Can. Biol. 31*:239–246, 1972.

Dement, W., Guilleminault, C., and Zarcone, V. Progress in clinical sleep research. Scientific exhibit at the American Medical Association, Atlantic City, June 14–18, 1975a.

Dement, W., Guilleminault, C., and Zarcone, V. The pathologies of sleep: A case series approach, in *The Nervous System*, Tower, D. H. (ed.), vol. 2 of *The Clinical Neurosciences*. Raven Press, New York, 1975b, pp. 501–517.

Dement, W. C., Carskadon, M. A., Mitler, M. M., Phillips, R. L., and Zarcone, V. P., Jr. Prolonged use of flurazepam: A sleep laboratory study. *Behav. Med.* October 1978, pp. 25–31.

Deneau, G. A., Yanagita, T., and Seevers, M. H. Self-administration of psycho-active substances by the monkey. *Psychopharmacologia* (Berlin) 16:30–48, 1969.

Derbez, R., and Grauer, H. A sleep study and investigation of a new hypnotic compound in a geriatric population. *Can. Med. Assoc. J.* 97:1388–1393, 1967.

Des Andres, I., Gutierrez-Rivas, E., Vava, E., and Reinoso-Suarez, F. Independence of sleep–wakefulness cycle in an implanted head "encephale-isole." *Neurosc. Lett.* 2:13–18, 1976.

de Silva, J. A. F., and Strojny, N. Determination of flurazepam and its major biotransformation products in blood and urine by spectrophotofluorometry and spectrophotometry. *J. Pharm. Sci.* 60:1303–1314, 1971.

Detre, T. Sleep disorder and psychosis. *Can. Psychiatr. Assoc. J.* 11:5169–5177, 1966.

Devenyi, P., and Wilson, M. Abuse of barbiturates in an alcoholic population. *Can. Med. Assoc. J.* 104:219–221, 1971.

Diamond, M. J., Brownstone, Y. S., Erceg, G., Kieraszewicz, H., and Keeri-Szanto, M. The reduction of coma time in lipophilic drug overdose using castor oil. *Can. Anaesth. Soc. J.* 23(2):170–175, 1976.

Dietze, V. F., Kalbe, I., Kranz, D., Brusckke, G., and Richter, H. Geriatrische Aspekte der Eisenresorption. *Z. Alternasforsch.* 24:229–235, 1971.

Domino, E. F., Yamamoto, K., and Dren, A. T. Role of cholinergic mechanisms in states of wakefulness and sleep. *Prog. Brain Res.* 28:113–133, 1968.

Dorfman, A., and Goldbaum, L. R. Detoxification of barbiturates. *J. Pharmacol. Exp. Ther.* 90:330–337, 1947.

Douglas, W. W. Histamine and antihistamines; 5-hydroxytryptamine and antagonists, in *The Pharmacological Basis of Therapeutics*, Goodman, L. S., and Gilman, A. (eds.), Macmillan, New York, 1975, pp. 590–629.

Dreisbach, R. H. Depressants, in *Handbook of Poisoning: Diagnosis and Treatment*, 9th ed. Lange Medical Publications, Los Altos, Calif., 1977, p. 310.

Drucker-Colín, R. R., and Spanis, C. W. Is there a sleep transmitter? *Prog. Neurobiol.* 6:1–22, 1976.

Drug Abuse Warning Network (DAWN), *Phase IV Report*, Drug Enforcement Administration, National Institute on Drug Abuse, BNDD Contract No. 72–47, 1976, pp. 1–203.

Dundee, J. W. Alterations in response to somatic pain associated with anaesthesia. II. The effect of theopentone and Pentobarbitone. *Br. J. Anaesth.* 32:407–414, 1960.

Dundee, J. W., Howard, A. J., and Isaac, M. Alcohol and the benzodiazepines: The interaction between intravenous ethanol and chlordiazepoxide and diazepam. *Q. J. Stud. Alcohol* 32:960–968, 1971.

Eckerman, W. C., Bates, J. D., Bachel, J. V., and Poole, W. K. Drug usage and arrest charges: A study of drug usage and arrest charges among arrestees in six metropolitan areas of the United States. Bureau of Narcotics and Dangerous Drugs, U.S. Department of Justice, Final Report, BNDD Contract No. J–70–35 (SCID–TR–4), Washington, D.C., 1971.

Eddy, N. B., Halbach, H., Isbell, H., and Seever, M. H. Drug dependence: Its significance and characteristics. *Psychopharmacol. Bull.* 3:1–12, 1966.

Ehrnebo, M. Pharmacokinetics and distribution properties of pentobarbital in humans following oral and intravenous administration. *J. Pharm. Sci.* 63:1114–1118, 1974.

Endrenyi, L., Inaba, T., and Kalow, W. Genetic study of amobarbital elimination based on its kinetics in twins. *Clin. Pharmacol. Ther.* 20:701–714, 1976.

Ertama, L., Honkanen, R., and Kuosmanen, P. Drugs as a risk factor in accidental falls. Abstracts, 7th International Conf. Pharmacol., Paris, 1978.

Essig, C. F., and Fraser, H. F. Electroencephalographic changes in man during use and withdrawal of barbiturates in moderate dosage. *Electroencephlogr. Clin. Neurophysiol.* 10:649–659, 1958.

Evans, D., and Bond, I. Reciprocal inhibition therapy and classical conditioning in the treatment of insomnia. *Behav. Res. Ther.* 7:315–316, 1969.

Ewart, R. B. L., and Priest, R. G. Methaqualone addiction and delirium tremens. *Br. Med. J.* 3:92–93, 1967.

Exton-Smith, A. N., Hodkinson, H. M., and Crowie, B. W. Controlled comparison of four sedative drugs in elderly patients. *Br. Med. J.*, October 1963, pp. 1037–1040.

Fabre, L. F., Gross, L., Pasagajen, V., and Metzler, C. Multiclinic double-blind comparison of triazoléum and flurazepam for seven nights in outpatients with insomnia. *J. Clin. Pharmacol.* 17:402–409, 1977.

Federal Register, 1975, Over-the-counter sleep-aid drug products, December 8, pp. 57292–57329.

Federal Register, 1978, Over-the-counter nighttime sleep-aid and stimulant products, June 13, pp. 25544–25602.

Feinberg, I., Hibi, S., Cavness, C., and March, J. Absence of REM rebound after barbiturate withdrawal. *Science* 185:534–535, 1974.

Feinberg, I., Fein, G., Walker, J. M., Price, L. J., Floyd, T. C., and March, J. D. Flurazepam effects on sleep EEG. *Arch. Gen. Psychiatry* 36:95–102, 1979.

Feinberg, S. M., and Bernstein, T. B. Histamine antagonists. *J. Lab. Clin. Med.* 32:1370–1373, 1947.

Feinberg, S., and Carlson, V. R. Sleep variable as a function of age in man. *Arch. Gen. Psychiatry* 18:239–250, 1968.

Fernandez, G., and Clarke, M. A case of "Veronal" poisoning. *Lancet*, 1:223–224, 1904.

Fillipini, L. Die Akut intermitterlude parphysie. *Intern. Praxis* 8:575–580, 1968.

Fingl, E., and Woodbury, D. M. General principles, in *The Pharmacological Basis of Therapeutics*, Goodman, L. S., and Gilman, A. (eds.), Macmillan, New York, 1975, pp. 1–46.

Finkle, B. S. Drugs in drinking drivers: A study of 2500 cases. *J. Saf. Res.* 1:179–183, 1969.

Fischer, H. D., and Oelssner, W. The influence of hexobarbital and phenobarbital on alcohol elimination in rabbits. *Med. Exp.* 3:213–218, 1960.

Fischer, H. D., and Oelssner, W. The effect of barbiturates on alcohol elimination in mice. *Klin. Wochenschr, 39:*1265, 1961.

Fishbein, W., and Gutwein, B. M. Paradoxical sleep and memory storage traces. *Behav. Biol.* 19:425–464, 1977.

Fischer, S., and Gal, P. Flurazepan versus amobarbital as a sedative–hypnotic for geriatric patients: Double-blind study. *J. Am. Geriatr. Soc.* 17(4):397–399, 1969.

Foulkes, D., Pivik, T., Aherns, J. G., and Swanson, E. M. Effects of dream deprivation on dream content: An attempted cross night replication. *Psychophysiology* 4:386–387, 1968.

Fowler, L. K. Temazepam (Euphypnos®) as a hypnotic: A twelve-week trial in general practice. *J. Int. Med. Res.* 5:295–296, 1977.

Fox, F. S. *Mythology of All Races*, vol. 1, Cooper Square Publishers, New York, 1964, p. 278.

Fracchia, J., Sheppard, C., Canale, D., Ruest, E., Cambria, E., and Merlis, S. Combination drug therapy for the psychogeriatric patient: Comparison of dosage levels of the same psychotropic drugs, used singly and in combination. *J. Am. Geriatr. Soc.* 23(11):508–511, 1975.

Frankel, B. L., Patten, B. M., and Gillin, J. C. Restless legs syndrome: Sleep-electro-encephalographic and neurologic findings. *J. Am. Med. Assoc. 230:*1302–1303, 1974.

Frankel, B. L., Coursey, R. D., Gaarder, K. R., and Mott, D. E. W. EMG biofeedback and autogenic training: Is either helpful in sleep-onset insomnia? *Sleep Res.* 4:215, 1975.

Frankel, B. L., Coursey, R. D., Buchbinder, R., and Snyder, F. Recorded and reported sleep in chronic primary insomnia. *Arch. Gen. Psychiatry 33:*615–623, 1976.

Fraser, H. F., and Jasinsky, D. R. The assessment of the abuse potentiality of seda-tive/hypnotics (depressants): Methods used in animals and man, in *Drug Addiction I,* Martin, W. R. (ed.), Springer-Verlag, New York, 1977, pp. 589–612.

Fraser, H. F., Wikler, A., Isbell, H., and Johnson, H. K. Partial equivalence of chronic alcohol and barbiturate intoxications. *Q. J. Stud. Alcohol 18:*541–551, 1957.

Fraser, H. F., Wikler, A., Essig, C. F., and Isbell, H. Degree of physical dependence induced by secobarbital of pentobarbital. *J. Am. Med. Assoc. 166:*126–129, 1958.

Freedman, R., and Papsdorf, J. D. Biofeedback and progressive relaxation treatment of sleep-onset insomnia: A controlled, allnight investigation. *Biofeedback and Self-Regulation 1:*253–271, 1976.

Freedman, R., Hauri, P., Coursey, R., and Frankel, B. Behavioral treatment of insomnia: A collaborative study. *Sleep Res.* 7:179, 1978.

Freeman, J., and Schulman, M. P. Reactions of chloral hydrate and ethanol with alcohol dehydrogenase for human liver. *Fed. Proc. Fed. Am. Soc. Exp. Biol.* 29:275, 1970.

Freemon, F. R. Clinical pharmacology of sleep in *Sleep Research: A Critical Review.* Charles C Thomas, Springfield, Ill., 1972, pp. 96–111.

Freemon, F. R. A critical review of all night polygraphic studies of sleeping medications, in *Hypnotics.* Kagan, F., Harwood, T., Rickels, K., Rudzik, A. D., and Sorer, H. (eds.),Spectrum, New York, 1975, pp. 41–56.

Freud, S. Project for a scientific psychology (1895), in *The Origins of Psychoanalysis: Letters to Wilhelm Fleiss, Drafts and Notes, 1887–1902,* Bonaparte, M., Freud, A., and Kres, E. (eds.), Basic Books, New York, 1954, p. 400.

Friedman, P. J., and Cooper, J. R. The role of alcohol dehydrogenase in the metabolism of chloral hydrate. *J. Pharmacol. Exp. Ther. 129:*373–376, 1960.

Frolkis, V. V., Bezrukov, V. V., and Sinitsky, V. N. Sensitivity of central nervous structures to humoral factors in aging. *Exp. Geront.* 7:185–194, 1972.

Fruensgaard, K. Withdrawal psychoses: A study of 30 consecutive cases. *Acta Psychiatr. Scand. 53:*105–118, 1976.

Garattini, S., Marcucci, F., Morselli, P. L., and Mussini, E. The significance of measuring blood levels of benzodiazepines, in *Biological Effects of Drugs in Relation to Their Plasma Concentration,* Davies, D. S., and Prichard, B. N. C. (eds.), University Park Press, Baltimore, 1973, pp. 211–225.

Geer, J. H., and Katkin, E. S. Treatment of insomnia using a variant of systematic desensitization: A case report. *J. Abnorm. Psychol.* 71:161–164, 1966.

Gelfand, M. C., Winchester, L. P., Knepshield, J. H., Hanson, K. M., Cohan, S. L., Strauch, B. S., Geoly, K. L., Kennedy, A. C., and Schreiner, G. E. Treatment of severe drug overdosage with charcoal hemoperfusion. *Trans. Am. Soc. Artif. Organs 23:*599–605, 1977.

General Practitioner Research Group, Sedation with a new non-barbiturate compound. *Practitioner 195:*366–368, 1965.

Gerald, M. C., and Schwirian, P. M. Nonmedical use of methaqualone. *Arch. Gen. Psychiatry 28:*627–631, 1973.

Gershon, E. S., and Liebowitz, J. H. Sociocultural and demographic correlates of affective disorders in Jerusalem. *J. Psychiat. Res.* 12:37–50, 1975.

Gessner, P. K. Effect of trichloroethanol and of chloral hydrate on the *in vivo* rate of disappearance of ethanol in mice. *Arch. Int. Pharmacodyn. Ther. 202*:392–401, 1973.

Gessner, P. K., and Cabana, B. E. The effect of ethanol on chloral hydrate hypnosis in mice. *Fedn. Proc. Fed. Am. Socs. Exp. Biol. 23*:348–360, 1964.

Gessner, P. K., and Cabana, B. E. Chloral alcoholate: Reevaluation of its role in the interaction between the hypnotic effects of chloral hydrate and ethanol. *J. Pharmacol. Exp. Ther. 156*:602–605, 1967.

Gibson, I. J. M. Barbiturate delirium. *Practitioner 197*:345–347, 1966.

Gillin, J. C., Mendelson, W. B., Sitaram, N., and Wyatt, R. J. The neuropharmacology of sleep and wakefulness. *Annu. Rev. Pharmacol. Toxicol. 18*:563–579, 1978.

Gillin, J. C., Duncan, W., Pettigrew, T. D., Frankel, B. L., and Snyder, F. Successful separation of depressed, normal and insomniac subjects by EEG sleep data. *Arch. Gen. Psychiatry 36*:85–90, 1979.

Glauser, F. L., Smith, W. R., Caldwell, A., Hoshiko, M., Dolan, G. S., Baer, H., and Olsher, N. Ethchlorvynol (Placidyl)-induced pulmonary edema. *Ann. Intern. Med. 84*(1):46–48, 1976.

Gold, E., Gordis, L., Tonascia, J., and Szklo, M. Increased risk of brain tumors in children exposed to barbiturates. *J. Natl. Cancer Inst. 61*:1031–1034, 1978.

Goldstein, L., Graedon, J., Willard, D., Goldstein, F., and Smith, R. R. A comparative study of the effects of methaqualone and glutethimide on sleep in male chronic insomniacs. *J. Clin. Pharmacol. 110*:258–268, 1970.

Goldstein, S. E., Birnbom, F., Lancee, W. J., and Darke, A. C. Comparison of oxazepam, flurazepam and chloral hydrate as hypnotic sedatives in geriatric patients. *J. Am. Geriatr. Soc. 26*:366–371, 1978.

Good, R. Frontalis muscle tension and sleep latency. *Psychophysiology 12*:465–467, 1975.

Gould, T., and Shideman, F. E. The *in vitro* metabolism of thiopental by a fortified, cell-free tissue preparation of the rat. *J. Pharmacol. Exp. Terap. 104*:427–439, 1952.

Greenberg, R. Dream interpretation insomnia. *J. Nerv. Ment. Dis. 144*:18–21, 1967.

Greenberg, R., and Pearlman, C. Delirium tremens and dreaming. *Am. J. Psychiatry 124*:133–142, 1967.

Greenblatt, D. J. Drug therapy of insomnia, in *Clinical Psychopharmacology*, Bernstein, J. G. (ed.), PSG Publishing, Littleton, Mass., 1978, pp. 27–39.

Greenblatt, D. J., and Koch-Weser, J. Clinical pharmacokinetics. *N. Engl. J. Med. 293*:702–705, 964–970, 1975.

Greenblatt, D. J., and Shader, R. I. Nonprescription psychotropic drugs, in *Pharmacology in the Practice of Medicine*, Jarvik, M. E. (ed.), Appleton-Century-Crofts, New York, 1977, pp. 345–357.

Greenblatt, D. J., and Shader, R. I. *Benzodiazepines in clinical practice*, Raven Press, New York, 1974.

Greenblatt, D. J., Shader, R. I., and Koch-Weser, J. Flurazepam hydrochloride. *Clin. Pharmacol. Ther. 17*:1–14, 1975.

Greenblatt, D. J., Allen, M. D., and Shader, R. I. Toxicity of high-dose flurazepam in the elderly. *Clin. Pharmacol. Ther. 21*:355–361, 1977.

Griesinger, W. Berliner medicinisch-psychologische Gesellschaft. *Arch. Psychiatr. Nervenkr. 1*:200–204, 1868.

Gross, M. M., Goodenough, D. R., Hastey, J., and Lewis, E. Experimental study of sleep in chronic alcoholics before, during and after four days of heavy drinking, with a non-drinking comparison. *Ann. N.Y. Acad. Sci. 215*:254–275, 1973.

Gross, M. M., Goodenough, D., Tobin, M., Halpert, E., Lepose, D., Perlstein, A., Sirota, M., Dibianco, J., Fuller, R., and Kishner, I. Sleep disturbances and hallucinations in the acute alcoholic psychoses. *J. Nerv. Ment. Dis. 142*:493–514, 1966.

Guile, L. A. Rapid habituation to chlordiazepoxide "Librium." *Med. J. Aust. 2*:56–57, 1963.

Guilleminault, C., and Dement, W. C., eds. *Sleep Apnea Syndromes.* Alan R. Liss, Inc., New York, 1978, pp. 1–390.

Guilleminault, C., Spiegel, R., and Dement, W. C. A propos des insomnies. *Confrontations psychiatriques 15:*151–172, 1977.

Gupta, R. C., and Kofoed, J. Toxicological statistics for barbiturates, other sedatives, and tranquillizers in Ontario: A ten-year study. *Can. Med. Assoc. J. 94:*863–865, 1966.

Guth, P. H. Physiologic alterations in small bowel function with age: The absorption of D-xylose. *Am. J. Dig. Dis. 13:*565–571, 1968.

Guttman, D. A survey of drug-taking behavior of the elderly. Natl. Instit. on Drug Abuse, Services Research Report, 1977, pp. 1–108.

Haacke, H., Johnsen, K., and Kolenda, K. Interaction of pentobarbital, dipehylhydantoin, and digitoxin with perfused guinea-pig liver. *Arzneim. Forsch. 26:*835–839, 1976.

Haefely, W., Kulcsar, A., Mohler, H., Pieri, P., and Schaffner, R. Possible involvement of GABA in central actions of benzodiazepines. *Adv. Biochem. Psychopharmacol. 14:*131–151, 1975.

Haffner, J. F. W., Bo, O., and Lunde, P. K. M. Alcohol and drug consumption as causal factors in road traffic accidents in Norway. *J. Traffic Med. 2:*52–56, 1974.

Hagenbucher, J. T., and Kleh, J. Treatment of insomnia in geriatric patients: Double blind study with methyprylon and pentabarbital. *J. Am. Geriatr. Soc. 10:*1038–1040, 1962.

Haider, I. A comparative trial of Mandarx and dechloralphenazone. *Br. J. Psychiatry 114:*465–468, 1968.

Haider, I., and Oswald, I. Effects of amylobarbitone and nitrazepam on the electrodermogram and other features of sleep. *Br. J. Psychiatry 118:*519–522, 1971.

Hakkinen, S. Traffic accidents and psychomotor test performance: A follow-up study. *Mod. Probl. Pharmacopsychiatry 11:*51–66, 1976.

Hall, R. C. W., and Joffe, J. R. Aberrant response to diazepam. A new syndrome. *Am. J. Psychiatry 129:*738–742, 1972.

Hamilton, E. *Mythology.* Mentor (New American Library), New York, 1961, pp. 106–108.

Hammond, E. C. Some preliminary findings on physical complaints from a prospective study of 1,064,004 men and women. *Am. J. Public Health 54:*11–23, 1964.

Harned, B. K., Hamilton, H. C., and Cole, U. U. The effect of the administration of sodium bromide to pregnant rats on the learning ability of the offspring. *J. Pharmacol. Ther. 82:*215–226, 1944.

Harris, T. H. Methaminodiazepoxide. *J. Am. Med. Assoc. 172:*1162–1163, 1960.

Hartmann, E. The effect of four drugs on sleep patterns in man. *Psychopharmacologia 12:*346–353, 1968.

Hartmann, E. Sleep requirement: Long sleepers, short sleepers, variable sleepers, and insomniacs. *Psychosomatics 14:*95–103, 1973.

Hartmann, E. *The Sleeping Pill,* Yale University Press, New Haven, 1978, pp. 162–178.

Hartmann, E., and Cravens, J. The effects of long-term administration of psychotropic drugs on human sleep. I. Methodology and the effects of placebo. *Psychopharmacologia 33:*153–167, 1973a.

Hartmann, E., and Cravens, J. The effects of long-term administration of psychotropic drugs on human sleep. VI. The effects of chlordiazepoxide. *Psychopharmacologia 33:*233–245, 1973b.

Hartmann, E., and Cravens, J. The effects of long term administration of psychotroic drugs on human sleep: V., The effects of chloral hydrate. *Psychopharmacologia 33:*219–232, 1973c.

Hartmann, E., Baekland, F., and Zwilling, G. R. Psychological differences between long and short sleepers. *Arch. Gen. Psychiatry 26:*463–468, 1972.

Hartmann, E., Orzack, M. H., and Branconnier, R. Deficits produced by sleep deprivation: Reversal of D- and L- amphetamine. *Sleep Res. 3:*151, 1974.

Hartz, S. C., Heinonen, O. P., Shapiro, S., Siskind, V., and Sloane, D. Antenatal exposure to meprobamate and chlordiazepoxide in relation to malformations, mental development, and childhood mortality. *N. Engl. J. Med. 292*:726–728, 1975.

Harvey, S. C. Hypnotics and sedatives, in *The Pharmacological Basis of Therapeutics*, Goodman, L. S., and Gillman, A. (eds.), Macmillan, New York, 1975, pp. 102–136.

Hauri, P. A case series of 141 consecutive insomniacs evaluated at the Dartmouth sleep lab. *Sleep Res. 5*:193, 1976.

Hauri, P. The sleep disorders, in *Current Concepts*. Scope Publication, New York, 1977, pp. 1–76.

Hauri, P., and Cohen, S. Treatment of insomnia with biofeedback: Final report of study 1. *Sleep Res. 6*:136, 1977.

Hauri, P. J., and Silberfarb, P. M. The effects of aspirin on the sleep of insomniacs. *Sleep Res. 7*:100, 1978.

Haynes, S., Follingstad, D., and McGowan, W. Insomnia: sleep patterns and anxiety level. *J. Psychosom. Res. 18*:69–74, 1974.

Hayes, S. L., Pablo, G., Radomski, T., and Palmer, R. F. Ethanol and oral diazepam absorption. *N. Engl. J. Med. 296*:186–189, 1977.

Haynes, S. N., Price, M. G., and Simons, T. B. Stimulus control treatment of insomnia. *J. Behav. Ther. Exp. Psychiatry 6*:279–282, 1975.

Hecht, A. Panel reports on sleep-aids. *FDA Consumer 10*:10–13, 1976.

Heider, F. *The Psychology of Interpersonal Relations*. Wiley, New York, 1958.

Held, H. Effect of alcohol on the heme and porphyrin synthesis: Interaction with phenobarbital and pyrayole. *Digestion 15*:136–146, 1977.

Hetland, L. B., and Couri, D. Effects of ethanol on glutethimide absorption and distribution in relationship to mechanism for toxicity enhancement. *Toxicol. Appl. Pharmacol. 30*:26–35, 1974.

Hill, H. E., Haertzen, C. A., and Yamahiro, R. S. The addict physician: A Minnesota Multiphasic Personality Inventory study of interaction of personality characteristics and availability of narcotics, in *The Addictive States*, Wikler, A. (ed.), Res. Publ. of the Assn. for Nerv. Ment. Dis., vol. 46, Williams and Wilkins, Baltimore, 1968, pp. 321–332.

Hill, R. M., Craig, J. P., Chaney, M. D., Tennyson, L. M., and McCulley, L. B. Utilization of over-the-counter drugs during pregnancy. *Clin. Obstet. Gynecol. 20*(2):381–394, 1977.

Hindmarch, I., Parrott, A. C., and Arerillas, L. A repeated dose comparison of dichloralphenazone, flunitrazepam and amylobarbitone sodium on some aspects of sleep and early morning behavior in normal subjects. *Br. J. Clin. Pharmacol. 4*:229–233, 1977.

Hinkle, J. E., and Lutker, E. R. Insomnia: A new approach. *Psychotherapy 9*:236–237, 1972.

Hinton, J. M. A comparison of the effects of six barbiturates and a placebo on insomnia and motility in psychiatric patients. *Br. J. Pharmacol. 20*:319–325, 1963.

Hirsch, C. S., Valentour, J. C., Adelson, L., and Sunshine, I. Unexpected ethanol in drug-intoxicated persons. *Postgrad. Med. 54*:53–57, 1973.

Hobson, J. A., McCarley, R. W., and McKenna, T. M. Cellular evidence bearing on the pontine brain-stem hypothesis of desynchronized sleep control. *Prog. Neurobiol.* (Oxford) *6*:280–376, 1976.

Hodes, B. Nonprescription drugs: An overview. *Int. J. Health Services 4*:125–130, 1974.

Hohenthal, T. T. Comparative clinical studies of a new somnifacient combination of methaqualone and etodioxine versus glutethimide and placebo. *Arzeniem. Forsch. 19*:1527–1529, 1969.

Holland, J., Marrie, M. J., Grant, C., and Plumb, M. M. Drugs ingested in suicide attempts and fatal outcome. *N.Y. State J. Med. 75*:2343–2349, 1975.

Hollister, L. E. Overdoses of psychotherapeutic drugs, in *Psychiatric Treatment: Crisis, Clinic and Consultation*, Rosenbaum, C. P., and Beebe, J. E. (eds.), McGraw-Hill, New York, 1975, pp. 145–154.

Hollister, L. E. Prescribing drugs for the elderly, *Geriatrics*, 32:71–73, 1977.

Hollister, L. E., Motzenbecher, F. P., and Degan, R. O. Withdrawal reactions from chlordiazepoxide "Librium." *Psychopharmacologia* 2:63–68, 1961.

Hollister, L. E., Bennett, J. L., Kimbell, I., Savage, L., and Overall, J. E. Diazepam in newly admitted schizophrenics. *Dis. Nerv. Syst.* 24:746–750, 1963.

Holloway, D. A. Drug problems in the geriatric patient. *Drug Intell. Clin. Pharm. 8:632–642,* 1974.

Houghton, G. W., Richens, A., Toseland, P. A., Davidson, S., and Falcover, M. A. Brain concentrations of phenytoin phenobarbitone and primidone in epileptic patients. *Eur. J. Clin. Pharmacol. 9:73–78,* 1975.

Hughes, F. W., Rountree, C. B., and Forney, R. B. Suppression of learned avoidance and discriminative responses in the rat by chlordiazepoxide (Librium) and ethanol–chlordiazepoxide combinations. *J. Genet. Psychol.* 103:139–145, 1963.

Hurd, E. P. *Sleep, Insomnia and Hypnotics.* George S. Davis, Detroit, 1891, pp. 89–112.

Hurwitz, N. Predisposing factors in adverse reactions to drugs. *Br. Med. J.* 1:536, 1969.

Inaba, D. S., Ray, G. R., Newmeyer, J. A., and Whitehead, C. Methaqualone abuse: Luding out. *J. Clin. Med. Assn. 224:* 1505–1509, 1973.

Inaba, T., and Kalow, W. Salivary excretion of amobarbital in man. *Clin. Pharmacol. Ther. 18:558–562,* 1975.

Inaba, T., Tang, B. K., Endrenyi, L., and Kalow, W. Amobarbital—a probe of hepatic drug oxidation in man. *Clin. Pharmacol. Ther. 20:439–444,* 1976.

Institute of Medicine. Sleeping pills, insomnia and medical practice. Report of a study by a Committee of the Institute of Medicine, 1979, pp. 1–198.

Irvine, R. E., Grove, J., Toseland, P. A., and Trounce, J. R. The effect of age on the hydroxylation of amylobarbitone sodium in man. *Br. J. Clin. Pharmacol. 1:41–43,* 1974.

Itil, T. M., Saletu, B., and Marasa, J. Determination of drug-induced changes in sleep quality based on digital computer "sleep prints." *Pharmakopsychiatr. Neuro-Psychopharmakol. 7:265–280,* 1974.

Jacobson, E. *Progressive Relaxation.* University of Chicago Press, Chicago, 1938.

Jacobson, E. *Anxiety and Tension Control.* J. B. Lippincott, Philadelphia, 1964.

Jensen, G. R. Addiction to "Noludar." *N. Z. Med. J. 59:431–432,* 1960.

Jetter, W. W., and McLean, R. Poisoning by the synergistic effect of phenobarbital and ethyl alcohol. *Arch. Pathol. 36:112–122,* 1943.

Jick, H. Comparative studies with hypnotic (RO 5-6901) under current investigation. *Curr. Ther. Res. Clin. Exp. 9(7):355–357,* 1967.

Johns, M. W., and Masterton, J. P. Effect of flurazepam on sleep in the laboratory. *Pharmacology 11:358–364,* 1974.

Johns, M. W., Gay, T. J. A., Masterton, J. P., and Bruce, D. W. Relationship between sleep habits, adrenocortical activity and personality. *Psychosom. Med. 33:499–508,* 1971.

Johnson, L. C. Psychological and physiological changes following total sleep deprivation, in *Sleep: Physiology and Pathology*, Kales, A. (ed.), J. B. Lippincott, Philadelphia, 1969, pp. 206–220.

Johnson L., and Clift, A. D. Dependence on hypnotic drugs in general practice. *Br. Med. J.* 4:613–617, 1968.

Johnson, L. C., Burdick, A., and Smith, J. Sleep during alcohol intake and withdrawal in the chronic alcoholic. *Arch. Gen. Psychiatry 22:406–418,* 1970.

Jones, B. E., Bobiller, P., Pin, C., and Jouvet, M. The effect of lesions of catecholamine-containing neurons upon monoamine content of the brain and EEG and behavioral waking in the cat. *Brain Res. 58:*157–177, 1973.

Jones, B. E., Harper, S. T., and Halaris, A. E. Effects of locus coeruleus lesions upon cerebral monoamine content, sleep–wakefulness states and the response to amphetamine in the cat. *Brain Res. 124:*473–496, 1977.

Jones, H. S., and Oswald, R. Two cases of healthy insomnia. *Electroencephalogr. Clin. Neurophysiol. 24:*378–380, 1968.

Jori, A. Potentiation of noradrenaline toxicity by drugs with antihistamine activity. *J. Pharm. Pharmacol. 18:*824, 1966.

Jouvet, M. Recherches sur les structures nerveuses et les méchanismes responsables des différentes phases du sommeil physiologique. *Arch. Ital. Biol. 100:*125–206, 1962.

Jouvet, M. Biogenic amines and the states of sleep. *Science 163:*32–41, 1969.

Jouvet, M. The role of monoamines and acetylcholine containing neurons in the regulation of the sleep–waking cycle. *Ergeb. Physiol. Biol. Chem. Exp. Pharmakol. 64:*166–307, 1972.

Jouvet, M., and Delorme, F. Locus coeruleus et sommeil paradoxal. *C. R. Soc. Biol. 159:*895–899, 1965.

Jouvet, M., and Michel, F. Correlations électromyographiques du sommeil chez le chat décortique et mésencephalique chronique. *C. R. Soc. Biol. 153:*422–425, 1959.

Joyce, C. R. B., Malpas, A., Rowan, J., and Scott, D. F. Behaviour and EEG are affected on the day after hypnotic doses of nitrazepam and amylobarbitone sodium. *Br. J. Pharmacol. 37:*503P–504P, 1969.

Kadar, D., Inaba, T., Endrenyi, L., Johnson, G. E., and Kalow, W. Comparative drug elimination capacity in man—glutethimide, amobarbital, antipyrine and sulfinpyrazone. *Clin. Pharmacol. Ther. 14:*552–560, 1974.

Kahn, M., Baker, B. L., and Weiss, J. M. Treatment of insomnia by relaxation training. *J. Abnorm. Psychol. 73:*556–558, 1968.

Kales, A., and Cary, G. Insomnia, evaluation and treatment in *Psychiatry* (suppl. to *Medical World News*), Robins, E. (ed.), 1971, pp. 55–56.

Kales, A., Hodemaker, F. S., Jacobson, A., and Lichtenstein, E. L. Dream deprivation: An experimental reappraisal. *Nature* (London) *204:*1337–1338, 1964.

Kales, A., Malmstrom, E. J., Scharf, M. B., and Rubin, R. T. Psychophysiological and biochemical changes following use and withdrawal of hypnotics, in *Sleep: Physiology and Pathology*, Kales, A. (ed.), J. B. Lippincott, Philadelphia, 1969, pp. 331–343.

Kales, A., Allen, C., Scharf, M. B., and Kales, J. D. Hypnotic drugs and their effectiveness. *Arch. Gen. Psychiatry 23*(3):226–232, 1970.

Kales, A., Kales, J. D., Scharf, M. B., and Tan, T. Hypnotics and altered sleep-dream patterns. II. All-night EEG studies of chloral hydrate, flurazepam, and methaqualone. *Arch. Gen. Psychiatry 23:*219–225, 1970.

Kales, A., Preston, T. A., Tan, T. L., and Allen, C. Hypnotics and altered sleep-dream patterns. I. All-night studies of glutethimide, methylprylon, and pentobarbital. *Arch. Gen. Psychiatry 23:*211–218, 1970.

Kales, A., Tan, T. L., Keller, E. J., Naitoh, P., Preston, T. A., and Malstrom, E. J. Sleep patterns following 205 hours of sleep deprivation. *Psychosom. Med. 32:*189–200, 1970.

Kales, A., Bixler, E. O., Leo, L. A., Healy, S., and Slye, E. Incidence of insomnia in the Los Angeles metropolitan area. *Sleep Res. 3:*139, 1974.

Kales, A., Bixler, E. O., Tan, T. L., Scharf, M. B., and Kales, J. D. Chronic hypnotic drug use: Ineffectiveness, drug-withdrawal insomnia, and dependence, *J. Am. Med. Assoc. 227:*513–517, 1974.

Kales, A., Kales, J. D., and Bixler, E. O. Insomnia, an approach to management and treatment. *Psychiatr. Annu. 4*(7):28–44, 1974.

Kales, A., Kales, J. D., Bixler, E. O., and Scharf, M. B. Effectiveness of hypnotic drugs with prolonged use: Flurazepam and pentobarbital. *Clin. Pharmacol. Ther.* 18(3):356–363, 1975.

Kales, A., Kales, J. D., and Humphrey, F. J. Sleep and dreams, in *Comprehensive Textbook of Psychiatry II*, Freedman, A. M., Kaplan, H. I., and Sadock, B. J. (eds.), Williams and Wilkins, Baltimore, 1975, pp. 114–128.

Kales, A., Bixler, E. O., Scharf, M., and Kales, J. D. Sleep Laboratory studies of flurazepam: A model for evaluating hypnotic drugs. *Clin. Pharmacol. Therap.* 576–583, 1976.

Kales, A., Hauri, P., Bixler, E. O., and Silberfarb, P. Effectiveness of intermediate-term use of secobarbital. *Clin. Pharmacol. Ther.* 20:541–545, 1976.

Kales, A., Kales, J. D., Bixler, E. O., Scharf, M. B., and Russek, E. Hypnotic efficacy of triazolam—sleep laboratory evaluations of intermediate-term effectiveness. *J. Clin. Pharmacol.* 16:399–406, 1976.

Kales, A., Bixler, E. O., Kales, J. D., and Scharf, M. B. Comparative effectiveness of nine hypnotic drugs: Sleep laboratory studies. *J. Clin. Pharacol.* 17:207–213, 1977.

Kales, A., Scharf, M. B., and Kales, J. D. Rebound insomnia: A new clinical syndrome. *Science* 201:1039–1041, 1978.

Kales, J., Kales, A., Bixler, E. O., and Slye, E. S. Effects of placebo and flurazepam on sleep patterns in insomniac subjects. *Clin. Pharmacol. Ther.* 12:691–697, 1971.

Kales, J., Tan, T., Swearingen, C., and Kales, A. Are over-the-counter sleep medications effective? All night EEG studies. *Curr. Ther. Res. Clin. Exp.* 13(3):143–151, 1971.

Kaplan, S. A., de Silva, J. A. F., Jack, M. L., Alexander, K., Strojny, N., Weinfeld, R. E., Puglisi, C. V., and Weissman, L. Blood level profile in man following chronic oral administration of flurazepam hydrochloride. *J. Pharm. Sci.* 62:1932–1935, 1973.

Karacan, I., Heine, W., Agnew, H. W., Williams, R. C., Webb, W. B., and Ross, J. J. Characteristics of sleep patterns during late pregnancy and the postpartum periods. *Am. J. Obstet. Gynecol.* 101(5):579–586, 1968.

Karacan, I., Williams, N. L., Finley, W. W., and Hursch, C. J. The effects of naps on nocturnal sleep: Influence on the need for stage 1 REM and stage 4 sleep. *Biol. Psychiatry* 2:391–399, 1970.

Karacan, I., Thornby, J. I., Anch, M., Holzer, C. E., Warheit, G. J., Schwab, J. J., and Williams, R. L. Prevalence of sleep disturbance in a primary urban Florida county. *Soc. Sci. Med.* 10:239–244, 1976.

Kato, R., Vassanelli, P., Frontino, K., and Chiesara, E. Variation in the activity of liver microsomal drug-metabolizing enzymes in rats in relation to age. *Biochem. Pharmacol.* 13:1037, 1964.

Kato, R., Takanaka, A., and Onoda, K-I. Studies on age differences in mice for the activity of drug-metabolizing enzymes of liver micromes. *Jpn. J. Pharmacol.* 20:572, 1970.

Kaul, A. F., Harsfield, J. C., Osathanondh, R., and Ostheimer, G. W. A retrospective analysis of analgesics and sedative–hypnotics in hospitalized obstetrical and gynecological patients. *Drug Intell. Clin. Pharm.* 12:95–99, 1978.

Kay, D. C., Blackburn, A. B., Buckingham, J. A., and Karacan, I. Human pharmacology of sleep, in *Pharacology of Sleep*, Williams, R. L., and Karacan, I. (eds.), John Wiley and Sons, New York, 1976, pp. 83–210.

Kay, D. C., Jasinski, D. R., Eisenstein, R. B., and Kelly, O. A. Quantified human sleep after pentobarbital. *Clin. Pharmacol. Ther.* 13:221–231, 1972.

Kehoe, J. P., and Abbott, A. P. Suicide and attempted suicide in the Yukon Territory. *Canad. Psychiatric Assn. J.* 20:15–23, 1975.

Kelley, H. Attribution theory in social psychology. *Nebraska Symposium on Motivation* 15:192–240, 1967.

Kellogg, R., and Baron, R. S. Attribution theory, insomnia, and the reverse placebo effect: A reversal of Storms' and Nisbett's findings. *J. Pers. Soc. Psychol.* 32:231–236, 1975.

Kelp, H. Chloral-wirkung in grossen dosen. *Allg. Z. Psychiatr. Ihre Grenzgeb.* 31:389–393, 1875.

Kennedy, P., Kreitman, N., and Ovenstone, I. M. The prevalence of suicide and parasuicide ('attempted suicide') in Edinburgh. *Brit. J. Psychiat.* 124:36–41, 1974.

Kesson, C. M., Gray, J. M. B., and Lawson, D. H. Benzodiazepine drugs in general medical patients. *Br. Med. J.* 1:680–682, 1976.

Khanna, J. M., and Kalant, H. Effect of inhibitors and inducers of drug metabolism on ethanol metabolism *in vivo. Biochem. Pharmacol.* 19:2033–2041, 1970.

Kirmil-Gray, K., Coates, T. J., Thoresen, C. E., Rosekind, M. R., and Price, V. A. Treating insomnia in adolescents. *Sleep Res.* 7:237, 1978.

Kleitman, N. *Sleep and Wakefulness.* University of Chicago Press, Chicago, 1963, pp. 208–212, 274, 341–350.

Klotz, U., Avant, G. R., Hoyumpa, A., Schenker, S., and Wilkinson, G. R. The effects of age and liver disease on the disposition and elimination of diazepam in adult man. *J. Clin. Invest.* 55:347–359, 1975.

Knowles, J. B., Laverty, S. G., and Kuechler, H. A. The effects of alcohol on REM sleep. *Q. J. Stud. Alcohol* 29:342–349, 1968.

Koch-Weser, J., and Sellers, E. M. Binding of drugs to serum albumin. *N. Engl. J. Med.* 294:311–316, 526–531, 1976.

Koff, R. S., Garvey, A. J., Burney, S. W., and Bell, B. Absence of an age effect on sulfobromophthalein retention in healthy men. *Gastroenterology* 65:300–302, 1973.

Kogan, H. *The Long White Line.* Random House, New York, 1963, pp. 85–102.

Korsgaard, S. Misbrug av lorazepam. *Vgeshrift for Laeger* 135:164–165, 1976.

Krafft-Ebing, R. V. Ueber Paraldehyde-Gebrauch und Missbrauch nebst einem Falle von Paraldehyde-Delirium. *Z. Ther.* 7:244, 1887.

Kramer, C. H. Methaqualone and chloral hydrate: Preliminary comparison in geriatric patients. *J. Am. Geriatr. Soc.* 15:455–461, 1967.

Kraus, J. Suicide behaviour in New South Wales. *Brit. J. Psychiat.* 126:313–318, 1975.

Kripke, D. F., Lavie, P., and Hernandez, J. Polygraphic evaluation of ethchlorvynol (14 days). *Psychopharmacology* 56:221–223, 1978.

Kripke, D. F., Simons, R. N., Garfinkel, L., and Hammond, E. C. Short and long sleep and sleeping pills. *Arch. Gen. Psychiatry* 36:103–116, 1979.

Kupfer, D. J., Wyatt, R. J., and Snyder, F. Comparison between electroencephalographic and systematic nursing observations of sleep in psychiatric patients. *J. Nerv. Ment. Dis.* 151:361–368, 1970.

Kupfer, D. J. REM latency: A psychobiologic marker for primary depressive diseases. *Biol. Psychiatry* 2:159–174, 1976.

Lasagna, L. A study of hypnotic drugs in patients with chronic diseases: Comparative efficacy of placebo, methyprylon (Noludar), meprobamate (Miltown, Equanil), pentobarbital, phenobarbital, secobarbital. *J. Chronic Dis.* 3:122–133, 1956.

Lawton, M. P., and Cahn, B. The effects of diazepam (Valium) and alcohol on psychomotor performance. *J. Nerv. Ment. Dis.* 133:550–554, 1963.

Leake, C. D. *An Historical Account of Pharmacology.* Charles C Thomas, Springfield, Ill., 1975, pp. 153–158.

Learoyd, B. M. Psychotropic drugs and the elderly patient. *Med. J. Aust.* 1:1131–1133, 1972.

LeBreton, R., and Garat, J. Suicides par les dérivés barbituriques associés à l'alcool ethylique. *Chrn. Med. Leg. (Paris)* 45:78–80, 1965.

Legendre, R., and Pieron, H. Des résultats histophysiologiques de l'injection intraoccipitoatlontoidedienne des liquides insomniques. *C. R. Soc. Biol. 68*:1108–1109, 1910.

Lehmann, H. E., and Ban, T. A. The effect of hypnotics on rapid eye movement (REM). *Int. Z. Klin. Pharmakol. Ther. Toxikol. 1*:424–427, 1968.

Lélek, I., and Danhauser, V. Experience with methaqualone (Motolon) sleep disorders. *Ther. Hung. 18*(1):31–32, 1970.

Lemere, F. Habit-forming properties of meprobamate. *Arch. Neurol. Psychiatry 76*:205–206, 1956.

Lenard, H. G., and Schulte, F. J. Polygraphic sleep study in craniopagus turns. *J. Neurol. Neurosurg. Psychiatry 35*:756–760, 1976.

Le Riche, W. H., and Csima, A. A clinical evaluation of four hypnotic agents, using a Latin-square design. *Can. Med. Assoc. J. 91*:435–438, 1964.

Le Riche, W. H., and Van Belle, G. Clinical and statistical evaluation of six hypnotic agents. *Can. Med. Assoc. J. 88*:837, 1963.

Le Riche, W. H., Csima, A., and Dobson, M. A clinical trial of four hypnotic drugs. *Can. Med. Assoc. J. 95*:300–302, 1966.

Lester, B. K., Rundell, O. H., Cowden, L. C., and Williams, H. L. Chronic alcoholism, alcohol and sleep. *Adv. Exp. Med. Biol. 35*:261–279, 1973.

Lick, J. R., and Heffler, D. Relaxation training and attention placebo in the treatment of severe insomnia. *J. Consult. Clin. Psychol. 45*:153–161, 1977.

Linet, O. I., and Rudzik, A. D. Comparison of triazolam and methyprylon as a hypnotic in insomniacs. *Psychopharmacol. Commun. 1*(5):473–480, 1975.

Linne, I. Attempted drug suicide in a Swedish city. *Acta Medica Scand. 195*:521–525, 1974.

Linnoila, M. Psychomotor effects of drugs and alcohol on healthy volunteers and psychiatric patients in *Advances in Pharmacology and Therapeutics, Vol. 8*, Olive, G. (ed.), Pergamon Press, New York, 1978.

Linnoila, M., and Mattila, M. J. Drug interaction on driving skills as evaluated by laboratory tests and by a driving simulator. *Pharmacopsychiatry 6*:127–132, 1973a.

Linnoila, M., and Mattila, M. J. Drug interaction on psychomotor skills related to driving: Diazepam and alcohol. *Eur. J. Clin. Pharmacol. 5*:186–194, 1973b.

Linnoila, M., and Viukari, M. Efficacy and side effects of nitrazepam and thioredazine as sleeping aids in psychogeratric inpatients. *Br. J. Psychiatry 128*:566–569, 1976.

Linnoila, M., Otterstrom, S., and Mattila, M. Serum chlordiazepoxide, diazepam, and thioridazine concentrations after the simultaneous ingestion of alcohol or placebo drink. *Ann. Clin. Res. 6*:4–6, 1974.

Linnoila, M., Saario, I., and Maki, M. Effect of treatment with diazepam or lithium and alcohol on psychomotor skills related to driving. *Eur. J. Clin. Pharmacol. 7*:337–342, 1974.

Linnoila, M., Saario, I., and Mattila, M. J. Drug–alcohol interaction on psychomotor skills during subacute treatment with benzodiazepines, flupenthixole, or lithium. *Br. J. Clin. Pharmacol. 1*:176, 1974.

Lomen, P., and Linet, O. I. Hypnotic efficacy of triazolam and methyprylon on insomniac inpatients. *J. Int. Med. Res. 4*(1):55–58, 1976.

Loennecken, S. J. *Acute Barbiturate Poisoning.* John Wright and Sons, Bristol, 1967, pp. 1–78.

Loomis, A. L., Harvey, E. N., and Hobart, G. A. Cerebral states during sleep, as studied by human brain potentials. *J. Exp. Psychol. 21*:127–144, 1937.

Lowery, C. R., Denney, D. R., and Storms, M. D. Insomnia: A comparison of the effects of placebo pill attributions and nonpejorative self-attributions. Unpublished manuscript, University of Kansas, 1976.

MacWilliam, J. A. Some applications of physiology to medicine. III. Blood pressure and heart action in sleep and dreams. *Br. Med. J. 2*:1196–1200, 1923.

Maggini, C., Murri, M., and Sacchatti, G. Evaluation of the effectiveness of temazepam on the insomnia of patients with neurosis and endogenous depression. *Arzneim. Forsch.* 19:1647–1652, 1969.

Maher, J. F., Schreiner, G. E., and Westervelt, F. B. Acute glutethimide intoxication. I. Clinical experience (22 patients) compared to acute barbiturate intoxication (63 patients). *Am. J. Med.* 33:70–82, 1962.

Malach, M., and Berman, N. Furosemide and chloral hydrate: Adverse drug interaction. *J. Am. Med. Assoc.* 232:638–639, 1975.

Malpas, A., Rowan, A. J., Joyce, C. R. B., and Scott, D. F. Persistent behavioural and electroencephalographic changes after single doses of nitrazepam and amylobarbitone sodium. *Br. Med. J.* 762–764, 1970.

Marchand, H. Über die Herbeiführung des bedingt-reflektorischen Schlafes ohne Medikamente. *Ote. Gesundhives* 9:1255–1266, 1954.

Margolin, S., Perlman, P., Villani, F., and McGauch, T. H. New class of hypnotics: Unsaturated carbinols. *Science* 144:384–385, 1951.

Mark, L. C. Pharmacokinetics of barbiturates, in *Acute Barbiturate Poisoning*, Matthew, H. (ed.). Excerpta Medica, Amsterdam, 1971, pp. 75–83.

Marley, E., and Vane, J. R. Tryptamine receptor in the central nervous system: Effects of anesthetics. *Nature* (London) 198:441–444, 1963.

Marshall, A. J. Cardiac arrhythmias caused by chloral hydrate. *Br. Med. J.* 150:994–995, 1977.

Marshall, E. K., and Owens, A. H. Absorption, excretion and metabolic fate of chloral hydrate and trichloroethanol. *Bull. Johns Hopkins Hosp.* 95:1–18, 1954.

Martilla, J. K., Hammel, R. J., Alexander, B., and Zustiak, R. Potential untoward effects of long-term use of flurazepam in geriatric patients. *J. Am. Pharm. Assoc.* 17(11):692–695, 1977.

Martin, W. R. General problems of drug abuse and drug dependence, in *Drug Addiction I*, Martin, W. R. (ed.), Springer-Verlag, New York, 1977, pp. 3–40.

Martin, Y. C. The effect of ethchlorvynol on the drug-metabolizing enzymes of rats and dogs. *Biochem. Pharmacol.* 16:2041–2044, 1967.

Matthew, H. Barbiturates. *Clin. Toxicol.* 8:495–513, 1975.

Matthew, H., and Lawson, A. A. H. Acute barbiturate poisoning: A review of two years' experience. *Q. J. Med.* 35:539–552, 1966.

Matthew, H., Proudfoot, A. T., Aitkin, R. C. B., Raeburn, J. A., and Wright, N. Nitrazepam—a safe hypnotic. *Br. Med. J.* 3:23–25, 1969.

Matthew, H., Roscoe, P., and Wright, N. Acute poisoning. *Practitioner* 208:254–258, 1972.

McGhie, A., and Russell, S. M. The subjective assessment of normal sleep patterns. *J. Ment. Sci.* 108:642–654, 1962.

McKenzie, R. E., and Elliott, L. L. Effects of secobarbital and D-amphetamine on performance during a simulated air mission. *Aerosp. Med.* 36:774–779, 1965.

McLeod, S. M., Giles, H. G., Patzalek, G., Thiessen, J. J., and Sellers, E. M. Diazepam actions and plasma concentrations following ethanol ingestion. *Eur. J. Clin. Pharmacol.* 11:345–349, 1977.

Meddis, R., Pearson, A., and Langford, G. An extreme case of healthy insomnia. *Electroencephalogr. Clin. Neurophysiol.* 35:213–214, 1973.

The Medical Letter on Drugs and Therapeutics. Interactions of alcohol with other drugs, 16:91–92, 1974.

The Medical Letter on Drugs and Therapeutics. Adverse interaction of drugs, 19:5–12, 1977.

Meech, R. W. Intracellular calcium injection causes increased potassium conductance in aplysia nerve cells. *Comp. Biochem. Physiol.* 424:493–499, 1972.

Melville, K. I., Joran, G. E., and Douglas, D. Toxic and depressant effects of alcohol given orally in combination with glutethimide or secobarbital. *Toxicol. Appl. Pharmacol. 9:*363–375, 1966.

Mellor, C. S., and Imlah, N. W. Hypnotic drug trial in dementia. *J. Ther. Clin. Res. 3:*9–11, 1966.

Mendelson, W. B. Pharmacologic and electrophysiological effects of ethanol in relation to sleep, in *Biochemistry and Pharmacology of Ethanol II,* Majchrowicz, E., and Noble, E. (eds.), Plenum Press, New York, 1979, pp. 467–483.

Mendelson, W. B., and Hill, S. Y. The effects of the acute administration of ethanol on the sleep of the rat: A dose-response study. *Pharmacol. Biochem. Behav. 8:*723–726, 1978.

Mendelson, W. B., Guthrie, R. D., Frederick, G., and Wyatt, R. J. The flower pot technique of rapid eye movement (REM) sleep deprivation. *Pharmacol. Biochem. Behav. 2:*553–556, 1974.

Mendelson, W. B., Reichman, J., and Othmer, E. Serotonin inhibition and sleep. *Biol. Psychiatry 10:*459–464, 1975.

Mendelson, W. B., Goodwin, D. W., Hill, S. Y., and Reichman, J. D. The morning after: Residual EEG effects on temazepam and flurazepam, alone and in combination with alcohol. *Curr. Ther. Res. Clin. Exp. 19:*155–163, 1976.

Mendelson, W. B., Gillin, J. C., and Wyatt, R. J. *Human Sleep and Its Disorders.* Plenum Press, New York, 1977, pp. 131–146.

Meyers, F. H., and Abreu, B. E. A comparison of the central and peripheral effects of atropine, scopalamine and some synthetic atropine-like compounds. *J. Pharmacol. Exp. Ther. 104:*387–395, 1952.

Mezey, E. Effect of phenobarbital administration on ethanol oxidizing enzymes and on rates of ethanol degradation. *Biochem. Pharmacol. 20:*508–510, 1971.

Miklovich, L., and van den Berg, B. J. Effects of prenatal meprobamate and chlordiazepoxide hydrochloride on human embryonic and fetal development. *N. Engl. J. Med. 291:*1268–1271, 1975.

Miller, A. I., D'Agostino, A., and Minsky, R. Effects of combined chlordiazepoxide and alcohol in man. *Q. J. Stud. Alcohol 24:*9–13, 1963.

Mishara, B. L., and Kastenbaum, R. Wine in the treatment of long-term geriatric patients in mental institutions. *J. Am. Geriatr. Soc. 22*(2):88–94, 1974.

Mitler, M., Phillips, R. L., Billiard, M., Spiegel, R., Zarcone, V., and Dement, W. C. Long-term effectiveness of temazepam 30mg H.S. on chronic insomniacs. *Sleep Res. 4:*109, 1975.

Mixing Mandrax and alcohol. *Br. Med. J. 2:*45, 1973.

Moeschlin, S. Clinical features of acute barbiturate poisoning, in *Acute Barbiturate Poisoning,* Matthew, H. (ed.). Excerpta Medica, Amsterdam, 1971.

Molander, L., and Duvhok, C. Acute effects of oxazepam, diazepam and methaqualone, alone and in combination with alcohol on sedation, coordination and mood. *Acta Pharmacol. Toxicol. 38:*145–160, 1976.

Monk, M., and Warchauer, M. E. Completed and attempted suicide in three ethnic groups. *Am. J. Epidemiol. 100:*333–345, 1974.

Monnier, M., Dudler, L., and Schoenenberger, G. A. Humoral transmission of sleep. VIII. Effects of the "Sleep Factor Delta" on cerebral motor, and visceral activities. *Pfuegers Arch. 345:*23–25, 1973.

Monnier, M., Dudler, L., Gaechter, R., Maier, P. F., Tobler, H. J., and Schoenenberger, G. A. The delta sleep inducing peptide (DSIP). Comparative properties of the original and synthetic nonapeptide. *Experientia 33:*548–552, 1977.

Monroe, L. J. Psychological and physiological differences between good and poor sleepers. *J. Abnorm. Psychol. 72:*255–264, 1967.

Morden, B., Conner, R., Mitchell, G., Dement, W., and Levine, S. Effects of rapid eye movement (REM) sleep deprivation on shock-induced fighting. *Physiol. Behav. 3:*425–432, 1968.

Morgan, H., Scott, D. F., and Joyce, C. R. B. The effects of four hypnotic drugs and placebo on normal subjects' sleeping and dreaming at home. *Br. J. Psychiatry 117:*649–652, 1970.

Morgan, H. F., Burns-Cox, C. J., Pocock, H., and Pottle, S. Deliberate self-harm: Clinical and socioeconomic characteristics of 368 patients. *Brit. J. Psychiat. 127:*564–574, 1975.

Morgane, P. J., and Stern, W. C. Chemical anatomy of brain circuits in relation to sleep and wakefulness. *Adv. Sleep Res. 1:*1–131, 1974.

Morland, J. Setekleiv, J., Haffner, J. F. W., Stromsaether, C. E., Danielsen, A., and Holst Wethe, G. Combined effects of diazepam and ethanol on mental and psychomotor functions. *Acta Pharmacol. Toxicol. 34:*5–15, 1974.

Morrison, D., and Mayfield, D. G. Sleep insurance: A valid use of hypnotics? *N.C. Med. J. 33:*862–865, 1972.

Moruzzi, G., and Magoun, H. W. Brain stem reticular formation and activation of the EEG. *Electroencephalogr. Clin. Neurophysiol. 1:*455–473, 1949.

Mould, G. P., Curry, S. H., and Binns, T. B. Interaction of glutethimide and phenobarbital with ethanol in man. *J. Pharm. Pharmacol. 24:*894–899, 1972.

Moxley III, J. H., Yingling, G. L., and Edwards, C. C. The Food and Drug Administration's over-the-counter drug review: Why review OTC drugs? *Fed. Proc. Fed. Am. Soc. Exp. Biol. 32*(4):1435–1437, 1973.

Muller, W., and Wollert, U. Interactions of benzodiazepines with serum albumin. Circular dichraism studies. *Naunyn Schmiedebergs Arch. Pharmacol. 278:*301–312, 1973.

Mulligan, A. F., and O'Grady, C. P. Reducing night sedation in psychogeriatric wards. *Nursing Times 67:*1089–1091, 1971.

Mullin, F. J., Kleitman, N., and Cooperman, N. R. Studies on the physiology of sleep. X. The effect of alcohol and caffeine on motility and body temperature during sleep. *Am. J. Physiol. 106:*478–487, 1933.

Murata, T. Metabolic fate of 1-ethynlcyclohexyl carbamate. II. Studies on the glucuronide excreted in the urine of humans receiving ethnylcychohexyl carbamate. *Chem. Pharm. Bull. 9:*146–149, 1961.

Murphy, G. E. The physician's responsibility for suicide. I. An error of commission. *Ann. Intern. Med. 82:*301–304, 1975a.

Murphy, G. E. The physician's responsibility for suicide. II. Errors of omission. *Ann. Intern. Med. 82:*305–309, 1975b.

Murphy, G. E. Suicide and attempted suicide. *Hosp. Pract.*, November 1977, pp. 73–81.

Murray, N. Methaminodiazepoxide, *J. Am. Med. Assoc. 173:*1760–1761, 1980.

Nagasaki, H., Iriki, M., Inone, S., and Vchizono, K. The presence of sleep-promoting material in the brain of sleep deprived rats. *Proc. Jpn. Acad. 50:*241–246, 1974.

Nair, N. P. V., and Schwartz, G. Triazolam in insomnia: A standard-controlled trial. *Curr. Ther. Res. Clin. Exp. 23:*388–392, 1978.

National Center for Health Statistics, Division of Vital Statistics, Mortality Statistics Branch. Data supplied by Mr. Don Greenberg.

National Disease and Therapeutic Index, conducted by IMS America, Ltd, 1977. All data cited appear in the following references: Institute of Medicine (1979) or NIDA Capsules (1978).

National Prescription Audit, conducted by IMS America, Ltd, 1977. All data cited appear in the following references: Institute of Medicine (1979) or NIDA Capsules (1978).

Nicassio, P., and Bootzin, R. A comparison of progressive relaxation and autogenic training as treatments for insomnia. *J. Abnorm. Psychol. 83:*253–260, 1974.

Nicolis, F. B. and Silvestri, L. G. Hypnotic activity of placebo in relation to severity of insomnia: A quantitative evaluation. *Clin. Pharm. Ther. 8*(6):841–848, 1967.

Nicoll, R. A. Pentobarbital: Action on frog motoneurons. *Brain Res. 94*:1–5, 1975a.

Nicoll, R. A. Presynaptic action of barbiturates in the frog spinal chord. *Proc. Natl. Acad. Sci. USA 72*:1460–1463, 1975b.

NIDA capsules: Top 26 problem drugs in the U.S. National Institute of Drug Abuse Publication C78–5A, May 1978.

Nimmo, W. S. Hypnotics, sedatives, tranquilizers and anitdepressants, in *Clinical Pharmacology*, Girdwood, R. H. (ed.), Ballière Tindall, London, 1976, pp. 169–193.

Nolan, N. A., and Parkes, M. W. The effect of benzodiazepines on the behavior of mice on a hole board. *Psychopharmacologia 29*:277–288, 1973.

Norheim, G. Abnormal drug distribution in fatal intoxications. *Forensic Sci. 3*:271–274, 1974.

O'Brien, J. P. Increase in suicide attempts by drug ingestion: Boston experience, 1964–1974. *Arch. Gen. Psychiat. 34*:1165–1169, 1974.

O'Connor, C. A., and Brodbin, P. A double-blind trial of the new hypnotic Mandrax. *Br. J. Clin. Pract. 21*:387–389, 1967.

Ogunremi, O. O., Adamson, L., Březinová, V., Hunter, W. M., Maclean, A. W., Oswald, I., and Percy-Robb, W. Two anti-anxiety drugs: A psychneuroendocrine study. *Br. Med. J. 2*:202–205, 1973.

O'Malley, K., Crooks, J., Duke, E., and Stevenson, I. H. Effect of age and sex on human drug metabolism. *Br. Med. J. 3*:607–609, 1971.

Opitz, J. M., Grosse, F. R., and Haneberg, B. Congenital effects of bromism? *Lancet 1*:91–92, 1972.

Orfanakis, N. G., and Galloway, W. B. Glutethimide poisoning. *Rocky Mount. Med. J. 74*(1):34, 1977.

Ostrenga, J. A. Editorial: Methaqualone—a Dr. Jekyll and Mr. Hyde? *Clin. Toxicol. 6*:607–609, 1973.

Oswald, I. Sleep mechanisms: Recent advances. *Proc. R. Soc.Med. 55*:910–912, 1962.

Oswald, I. The why and how of hypnotic drugs. *Brit. Med. J. 1*:1167–1168, 1979.

Oswald, I., and Priest, R. G. Five weeks to escape the sleeping pill habit. *Br. Med. J. 2*:1093–1099, 1965.

Oswald, I., Thacore, V. R., Adam, K., Brezinova, V., and Burack, R. Alpha-adrenergic receptor blockage increases human REM sleep. *Br. J. Clin. Pharmacol. 2*:107–110, 1975.

Overland, E. S., and Severinghaus, J. W. Noncardiac pulmonary edema. *Adv. Intern. Med. 23*:307–326, 1978.

Over-the-counter sleep-aid drug products. *Fed. Reg.*, December 8, 1975, pp. 57292–57329.

Over-the-counter nighttime sleep-aid and stimulant products. *Fed. Reg.*, June 13, 1978, pp. 25544–25602.

Owen, M., and Bliss, E. L. Sleep loss and cortical excitability. *Am. J. Physiol. 218*:171–173, 1970.

P'an, S. Y., Gardocki, J. F., Harfenist, M., and Bauley, A. Pharmacology of vinyl ethynl carbinols, a new class of central nervous system depressants. *J. Pharmacol. Exp. Ther. 107*:459–463, 1953.

Pappenheimer, J. R., Koski, G., Finch, V., Karnovsky, M. L., and Krueger, J. Extraction of sleep-promoting factor S from cerebrospinal fluid and from brains of sleep-deprived animals. *J. Neurophysiol. 38*:1299–1311, 1975.

Parke, D. V. Biochemistry of the barbiturates, in *Acute Barbiturate Poisoning*, Matthew, H. (ed.), Excerpta Medica, Amsterdam, 1971, pp. 7–53.

Parloff, M. B., Wolfe, B., Hadley, S., and Waskow, I. E. Assessment of psychosocial treatment of mental disorders: Current status and prospects. An invited paper of the Advisory Committee on Mental Health, Institute of Medicine, National Academy of Sciences, submitted to the President's Commission on Mental Health, February 1978, pp. 1–324.

Parry, H. S., Balter, M. B., Mellinger, G. D., Cisin, I. H., and Manheimer, D. I. National patterns of psychotherapeutic drug use. *Arch. Gen. Psychiatry 28:*769–783, 1973.

Pathy, M. S. A double-blind comparison of chlormethiazole and dichloralphenazone: A sedative/hypnotic in geriatric medicine. *Curr. Med. Res. Opinion 2:*648–656, 1975.

Patrick, M. J., Tilstone, W. J., and Reavey, P. Diazepam and breast feeding. *Lancet 1:*542–543, 1972.

Pattison, J. H., and Allen, R. P. Comparison of the hypnotic effectiveness of secobarbital, pentobarbital, methyprylon and ethchlorvynol. *J. Am. Geriatr. Soc. 20*(8):398–402, 1972.

Pearlman, C., and Becker, M. REM sleep deprivation impairs bar-press acquisition in rats. *Physiol. Behav. 13:*813–817, 1974.

Pemberton, M. Use of phenylbutazone in rheumatoid arthritis. *Br. Med. J. 1:*490, 1954.

Perkins, R., and Hinton, J. Sedative or tranquillizer? A comparison of the hypnotic effects of chlordiazepoxide and amylobarbitone sodium. *Br. J. Psychiatry 124:*435–439, 1974.

Petersen, D. M., and Chambers, C. D. Demographic characteristics of emergency room admissions of acute drug reactions. *Int. J. of the Addictions 10:*963–975, 1975.

Petersen, H., and Brosstad, F. Pattern of acute drug poisoning in Oslo. *Acta Med. Scand. 201:*233–237, 1977.

Physical dependence on benzodiazepines? *Drug Ther. Bull. 15:*85–86, 1977.

Pines, A., Rooney, J. F. F., and Arenillas, L. Flurazepam (Dalmane) in the treatment of insomnia in patients with respiratory disorders. *Practitioner 217:*281–284, 1976.

Pokorny, A. D. Suicide rates in various psychiatric disorders. *J. Nerv. Ment. Dis. 139:*499–506, 1964.

Polc, P., Schneeberger, J., and Haefely, W. Effect of the delta sleep inducing peptide (DSIP) on the sleep-wakefulness cycle of cats. *Neurosci. Lett. 9:*33–36, 1978.

Pollack, C. P., McGregor, P., and Weitzman, E. The effects of flurazepam on daytime sleep after acute sleep–wake cycle reversal. *Sleep Res. 5:*112, 1975.

Pollard, H., Bischoff, S., and Schwartz, J. C. Decreased histamine synthesis in the rat brain by hypnotics and anaesthetics. *J. Pharm. 25:*920–927, 1973.

Pollard, H., Bischoff, S., and Schwartz, J. C. Turnover of histamine in rat brain and its decrease under barbiturate anaesthesia. *J. Pharmacol. Exp. Ther. 190:*88–90, 1974.

Polzella, P. J. Effects of sleep deprivation on short-term recognition memory. *J. Exp. Psychol. 104:*194–200, 1975.

Poser, E. G., Fenton, G. W., and Scotton, L. The classical conditioning of sleep and wakefulness. *Behav. Res. Ther. 3:*259–264, 1965.

Powell, W. F., and Comer, W. H. Double-blind controlled comparison of lorazepam and glutethimide in night before operation hypnotics. *Anesth. Analg. (Cleveland) 52:*313–316, 1973.

Price, V. A., Coates, T. J., Thoresen, C. E., and Grinstead, O. A. The prevalence and correlates of poor sleep among adolescents. *Am. J. Dis. Child. 132:*583–586, 1978.

Product Marketing: Consumer Expenditure Study, Supplement. July 1978a, pp. c–j.

Product Marketing: Marketing Emphasis. September 1978b, p. 89.

Quastel, J. H. Effects of drugs on energy metabolism of the brain and on cerebral transport, in *Handbook of Psychopharmacology,* vol. 5, Iversen, L. L., Iverson, S. D., and Snyder, S. H. (eds.), Plenum Press, New York, 1975, pp. 1–46.

Rada, R. T., Kellner, R., and Buckanan, J. G. Chlordiazepoxide and alcohol: A fatal overdose. *J. Forensic Sci. 20:*544–547, 1975.

Rado, S. The psychoanalysis of pharmacothymia (drug addiction). *Psychoanal. Q. 2:*1–23, 1933.

Randall, L. O., and Kappell, B. Pharmacological activity of some benzodiazepines and their metabolites, in *The Benzodiazepines,* Garattini, S., Mussini, E., and Randall, L. O. (eds.), Raven Press, New York, 1973, pp. 27–51.

Randall, L. O., Schallek, W., Heise, G. A., Keith, E. F., and Bagdon, R. E. The psychosedative properties of metbaminodiazepoxide. *J. Pharmacol. Exp. Ther. 129:*163–171, 1960.

Randall, L. O., Heise, G. A., Schallek, W., Bagdon, R. E., Bauziger, R. F., Boris, A., Moe, R. A., and Abrams, W. B. Pharmacological and clinical studies on Valium, a new psychotherapeutic agent of the benzodiapine class. *Am. Ther. Res. 3:*405–425, 1961.

Randall, L. O., Schallek, W., Scheckel, C. L., Stefko, P. L., Banziger, R. F., Pool, W., and Moe, R. A. Pharmacological studies on flurazepam hydrochloride (RO 5-6901) a new psychotropic agent of the benzodiazepine class. *Arch. Int. Pharmacodyn. Ther. 178:*216–241, 1969.

Rao, S., Sherbaniuk, R. W., Prosad, K., Lee, J. K., and Sproule, B. J. Cardiopulmonary effects of diazepam. *Clin. Pharmacol. Ther. 14:*182–189, 1973.

Raskin, M., Johnson, G., and Rondestvedt, J. Chronic anxiety treated by feedback-induced muscle relaxation: A pilot study. *Arch. Gen. Psychiatry 28:*263–266, 1973.

Rechtschaffen, A. Polygraphic aspects of insomnia, in *The Abnormalities of Sleep in Man*, Gastant, H., Lugaresi, E., Cerone, G. B., and Coccagna, G. (eds.), Anlo Gaggi, Bologna, 1969, pp. 109–125.

Rechtschaffen, A., and Kales, A. A manual of standardized terminology, techniques and scoring system for sleep stages of human subjects. Brain Information Service/Brain Research Institute, Los Angeles, 1968.

Rechtschaffen, A., Wolpert, E. A., Dement, W. C., Mitchell, S. A., and Fisher, C. Nocturnal sleep of narcoleptics. *Electroencephalogr. Clin. Neurophysiol. 15:*599–609, 1963.

Reed, C. E., Driggs, M. F., and Foote, C. C. Acute barbiturate intoxication: A study of 300 cases based on physiologic system of classification of severity of intoxication. *Ann. Intern. Med. 37:*290–303, 1952.

Reeves, R. L. Comparison of Triazolam, flurazepam, and placebo as hypnotics in geriatric patients with insomnia. *J. Clin. Pharmacol. 17:*319–323, 1977.

Ribordy, S. C., and Denney, D. R. The behavioral treatment of insomnia: An alternative to drug therapy. *Behav. Res. Ther. 15:*39–50, 1977.

Richey, D. P. Effects of human aging on drug absorption and metabolism, in *The Physiology and Pathology of Human Aging*, Goldman, R., and Rockstein, M. (eds.), Academic Press, New York, 1975, pp. 59–93.

Richter, E., Zilly, W., and Brachtel, D. Zur Frage der Barbiturattoleranz bei Patienten mit akuter Hepatitis. *Dtsch. Med. Wochenschr. 97:*254–255, 1972.

Rickels, K., and Bass, H. A comparative controlled clinical trial of seven hypnotic agents in medical and psychiatric inpatients. *Am. J. Med. Sci. 245:*142–152, 1963.

Reidenberg, M. M., Lowenthal, D. T., Briggs, W., and Gasparo, M. Pentobarbital elimination in patients with poor renal function. *Clin. Pharmacol. Ther. 20:*67–71, 1976.

Reider, J., and Wendt, G. Pharmacokinetics and metabolism of the hypnotic nitrazepam, in *The Benzodiazepines*, Garattini, S., Mussini, E., and Randall, L. O. (eds.), Raven Press, New York, 1973, pp. 99–127.

Risberg, A. M., Risberg, J., Elmquist, D., and Ingvar, D. H. Effects of dixyrazine and methaqualone on the sleep pattern in normal man. *Eur. J. Clin. Pharmacol. 8:*227–231, 1975.

Ritchie, J. M. The aliphalic alcohols, in *The Pharmacological Bases of Therapeutics*, Goodman, L. S., and Gilman, A. (eds.), Macmillan, New York, 1975, pp. 137–151.

Rosenlof, R. C., and Grissom, R. L. Clinical studies on a new nonbarbiturate sedative, ethyl-beta-chlorovinyl ethinyl carbinol (Placedyl). *Am. Pract. Dig. Treat. 8:*246–249, 1957.

Rosenbaum, J. L., Kramer, M. S., Raja, R., Winsten, S., and Dalal, F. Hyperfusion for acute drug intoxication. *Kidney Int. 10:*S341–S342, 1976.

Rosenthal, R., and Brown, J. M. Placidyl and pulmonary effects. *Ann. Intern. Med. 85:*126, 1976.

Ross, L., Rodin, J., and Zimbardo, P. G. Toward an attribution therapy: The reduction of fear through induced cognitive-emotional misattribution. *J. Pers. Soc. Psychol.* 12:279–288, 1969.

Roth, T., and Kramer, M. The nature of insomnia: A descriptive summary of a sleep clinic population. *Sleep Res.* 4:234, 1975.

Roth, T., Kramer, M., Leston, W., and Lutz, T. The effects of sleep deprivation on mood. *Sleep Res.* 3:154, 1974.

Rudolf, M., Geddis, D. M., Turner, J. A. McM., and Saunders, K. B. Depression of central respiratory drive by nitrazepam. *Thorax* 33:97–100, 1978.

Ruedy, J. Acute drug poisoning in the adult. *Can. Med. Assoc. J.* 109:603–608, 1973.

Saario, I., and Linnoila, M. Effect of subacute treatment with hypnotics, alone or in combination with alcohol, on psychomotor skills related to driving. *Acta Pharmacol. Toxicol.* 38:382–892, 1976.

Saario, I., Linnoila, M., and Maki, M. Interaction of drugs with alcohol on human psychomotor skills related to driving: Effect of sleep deprivation or two weeks' treatment with hypnotics. *J. Clin. Pharmacol.* 15:52–59, 1975.

Safra, M. J., and Oakley, G. P. Association between cleft lip with or without cleft palate and prenatal exposure to diazepam. *Lancet* 2:478–540, 1975.

Sagales, T., and Erill, S. Effects of central dopaminergic blockage with pimozide upon the EEG stages of sleep in man. *Psychopharmacologia* 41:53–56, 1975.

Sagales, T., Erill, S., and Domino, E. Differential effects of scopolamine and chlorpromazine on REM and NREM sleep in normal male subjects. *Clin. Pharmacol. Ther.* 10:522–529, 1969.

Salkind, M. R., and Silverstone, T. A clinical and psychometric evaluation of flurazepam. *Br. J. Clin. Pharmacol.* 2:223–226, 1975.

Sapienza, P. L. A double-blind comparison of methaqualone, pentobarbital and placebo in the management of insomnia. *Curr. Ther. Res. Clin. Exp.* 8(11):523–527, 1966.

Saxen, I. Associations between oral clefts and drugs taken during pregnancy. *Int. J. Epidemiol.* 4:37–44, 1975.

Schallek, K. W., Lewinson, T., and Thomas, J. Power spectrum analysis as a tool for statistical evaluation of drug effects on electrical activity of brain. *Int. J. Neuropharmacol.* 7:35–46, 1968.

Schenkel, B., and Vorherr, H. Non-prescription drugs during pregnancy: Potential teratogenic and toxic effects upon embryo and fetus. *J. Reprod. Med.* 12:27–45, 1974.

Schoenberg, B. S. Richard Caton and the electrical activity of the brain. *Mayo Clin. Proc.* 49:474–481, 1974.

Schultz, J. Adenosine 3′, 5-mono-phosphate in guinea pig cerebral cortical slices: Effect of benzodiazepines. *J. Neurochem.* 22:685–690, 1974a.

Schultz, J. Inhibition of phosphodieserase activity in brain cortical slices from guinea pig and rat. *Pharmacol. Res. Commun.* 6:335–341, 1974b.

Schwartz, M. A., and Postma, E. Metabolism of flurazepam, a benzodiazepine, in man and dog. *J. Pharm. Sci.* 59:1800–1806, 1970.

Schweiger, M. S. Sleep disturbance in pregnancy: A subjective survey. *Am. J. Obstet. Gynecol.* 114:(7):879–882, 1972.

Seeman, P. The membrane expansion theory of anesthesia, in *Progress in Anesthesiology, vol. 1, Molecular Mechanisms of Anesthesia*, Frich, B. R. (ed.), Raven Press, New York, 1975, pp. 243–252.

Seguin, E. C. The abuse and use of bromides. *J. Nerv. Ment. Dis.* 4:445–462, 1877.

Seidl, L. G., Thornton, G. F., Smith, J. W., and Cluff, L. E. Studies on the epidemiology of adverse drug reactions. III. Reactions in patients on a general medical service. *Bull. Johns Hopkins Hosp.* 119:299, 1966.

Selig, J. W. A possible oxazepam abstinence syndrome. *J. Am. Med. Assoc.* 198:279–280, 1966.

Sellers, E. M., and Koch-Weser, J. Kinetics and clinical importance of displacement of warfarin from albumin by acidic drugs. *Ann. N.Y. Acad. Sci. 179*:213–225, 1971.

Setter, J. G., Maher, J. F., and Schreiner, G. E. Barbiturate intoxication evaluation of therapy including analysis. *Arch. Intern. Med. 117*:224–236, 1966.

Shah, M. N., Clancy, B. A., and Iber, F. L. Comparison of blood clearance of ethanol and tolbutamide and activity of hepatic ethanol-oxidizing and drug-metabolizing enzymes in chronic alcoholic subjects. *Am. J. Clin. Nutr. 25*:135–139, 1972.

Shapiro, S., Slone, D., Lewis, G. P., and Jick, H. Clinical effects of hypnotics. *J. Am. Med. Assoc. 209*(13):2016–2020, 1969.

Sharpless, S. K. Hypnotics and sedatives, in *The Pharmacological Basis of Therapeutics*, Goodman, L. S., and Gilmer, A. (eds.), Macmillan, New York, 1965, p. 133.

Sherwin, A. L., Eisen, A. A., and Sokolowski, C. D. Anticonvulsant drugs in human epileptogenic brain. *Arch. Neurol. (Chicago) 29*:73–77, 1973.

Shubin, H., and Weil, M. H. The mechanism of shock following suicidal doses of barbiturates, narcotics and tranquilizer drugs, with observations on the effects of treatment. *Am. J. Med. 38*:853–863, 1965.

Shultz, J. H., and Luthe, W. *Autogenic Training*. Grune and Stratton, New York, 1959.

Siegel, J. M., and McGinty, D. J. Positive reticular formation neurons: Relationship of discharge to motor activity. *Science 196*:678–680, 1977.

Sievers, M. L., Cynamon, M. H., and Bittker, T. E. Intentional isoniazid overdosage among southwestern American Indians. *Am. J. Psychiat. 132*:423–428, 1975.

Sitaram, N., Wyatt, R. J., Dawson, S., and Gillin, J. C. REM sleep induction by physostigmine infusion during sleep in normal volunteers. *Science 191*:1281–1283, 1976.

Sjögen, J., Sövell, L., and Karlsson, I. Studies on the absorption rate of barbiturates in man. *Acta Med. Scand. 178*:553–559, 1965.

Slater, P. E., and Kastenbaum, R. Paradoxical reactions to drugs: Some personality and ethnic correlates. *J. Am. Geriatr. Soc. 14*(10):1016–1034, 1966.

Smith, C. M. The pharmacology of sedative/hypnotics, alcohol and anesthetics: Sites and mechanisms of action, in *Drug Addiction I*, Martin, W. R. (ed.), Springer-Verlag, New York, 1977, pp. 413–587.

Smith, D. E., and Wesson, D. R. Diagnosis and treatment of adverse reactions to sedative–hypnotics. NIDA, ADAMHA, USDHEW, 1974, pp. 1–68.

Smith, G. M., Coletta, C. G., McBride, S., and McPeek, B. Use of subjective responses to evaluate efficacy of mild analgesic-sedative combinations. *Clin. Pharmacol. Ther. 15*(2):118–129, 1974.

Smith, J. A., and Renshaw, D. C. A clinical study of insomnia. *Am. Fam. Physician/GP 11*:140–141, 1975.

Smith, J. W., Seidl, L. G., and Cluff, L. E. Studies on the epidemiology of adverse drug reactions: Five clinical factors influencing susceptibility. *Ann. Intern. Med. 65*(4):629, 1966.

Smith, J. W., Johnson, L. C., and Burdick, J. A. Sleep, psychological and clinical changes during alcohol withdrawal in NAD-tested alcoholics. *Q. J. Stud. Alcohol 32*:982–994, 1971.

Smith, R. B., Dittert, L. W., Griffen, W. O., Jr., and Doluisio, J. T. Pharmacokinetics of pentobarbital after intravenous and oral administration. *J. Pharmacokinet. Biopharm. 1*:5–16, 1973.

Snyder, F. The new biology of dreaming. *Arch. Gen. Psychiatry 8*:381–391, 1963.

Snyder, F. Dynamic aspects of sleep disturbance in relation to mental illness. *Biol. Psychiatry 1*:119–130, 1969.

Soehring, K., and Schuppel, R. Interactions between alcohol and drugs, in *Alcohol and Alcoholism*, Papharm, R. E. (ed.), University of Toronto Press, Toronto, 1970, p. 73.

Stern, F. H. Sleep-inducing properties of a nonbarbiturate analgesic/sedative preparation in elderly patients. *Clin. Med. 79*:31–33, 1972.

Stern, L., Khanna, N. N., Levy, G., and Yaffe, S. J. Effect of phenobarbital on hyperbilimbinemia and glucuronide formation in newborns. *Am. J. Dis. Child. 120*:26–31, 1970.

Stern, W. C. The relationship between REM sleep and learning: Animal studies, in *Sleep and Dreaming*, Hartmann, E. (ed.), Little, Brown and Co., Boston, 1970, pp. 225–249.

Sternbach, L. H., and Reeder, E. Quinazolines and 1,4-benzodiazephines. II. The rearrangement of 6-chloro-2-chloromethyl-4-phenzlquinazoline-3-oxide into 2-amino derivatives of 7-chloro-5-phenyl-3H-1,4-benzodiazepine 4-oxide. *J. Org. Chem. 26*:1111–1118, 1961.

Steinmark, S. W., and Borkovec, T. D. Active and placebo treatment effects on moderate insomnia under counterdemand and positive demand instructions. *J. Abnorm. Psychol. 83*:157–163, 1974.

Stolley, P. D., Becker, M. H., Lasagna, L., McEvilla, J. D., and Sloane, L. M. The relationship between physician characteristics and prescribing appropriateness. *Medical Care 10*:17–28, 1972.

Storms, M. D., and Nisbett, R. E. Insomnia and the attribution process. *J. Pers. Soc. Psychol. 16*:319–328, 1970.

Stotsky, B. A., Cole, J. O., Tang, Y. T., and Gahm, I. G. Sodium butabarbital (butisol sodium) as an hypnotic agent for aged psychiatric patients with sleep disorders. *J. Am. Geriatr. Soc. 19*:860–870, 1971.

Straus, B., Eisenberg, J., and Gennis, G. Hypnotic effects of an antihistamine—methapyrilene hydrochloride. *Ann. Intern. Med. 42*:574–582, 1955.

Streicher, E., and Garbus, J. The effect of age and sex on the duration of hexobarbital anesthesia in rats. *J. Gerontol. 10*:441–444, 1955.

Stuss, D., Healey, T., and Broughton, R. Personality and performance measures in natural extreme short sleepers. *Sleep Res. 4*:204, 1975.

Subcommittee on Long Term Care of the Special Committee on Aging, United States Senate. *Nursing Home Care in the United States: Failure in Public Policy*, Introductory Report. U. S. Government Printing Office, Washington, D. C., 1974.

Sunshine, A. A comparative study of Excedrin P.M. and placebo. *J. Clin. Pharmacol. 14*:166–171, 1974.

Sunshine, A. Comparison of the hypnotic activity of triazolam, flurazepam, hydrochloride, and placebo. *Clin. Pharmacol. Ther. 17*(5):573–577, 1975.

Svensmark, O., and Buchthal, F. Accumulation of phenobarbital in man. *Epilepsia 4*:199–206, 1963.

Swanson, D. W., Weddige, R. L., and Morse, R. M. Abuse of prescription drugs. *Mayo Clin. Proc. 4*:359–367, 1973.

Sweetwood, H. L., Kripke, D. F., Grant, I., Yager, J., and Gerst, M. S. Sleep disorder and psychobiological symptomatology in male psychiatric outpatients and male nonpatients. *Psychosom. Med. 38*:373–378, 1976.

Tansella, M., Zimmermann-Tansella, C., and Lader, M. The residual effects of N-desmethyldaizepam in patients. *Psychopharmacologia 38*:81–90, 1974.

Tansella, M., Siciliani, O., Burti, L., Schiavon, M., and Zimmermann-Tansella, C. N-desmethyldiazepam and amylobarbitone sodium as hypnotics in anxious patients: Plasma levels, clinical efficacy and residual effects. *Psychopharmacologia 41*:81–85, 1975.

Task Force on Prescription Drugs. *Final Report*. USDHEW, Washington, D. C., 1969, p. 2.

Tatum, A. L. The present status of the barbiturate problem. *Physiol. Rev. 19*:472–502, 1939.

Taylor, K. M., and Laverty, R. The interaction of chlordiazepoxide, diazepam, and nitrazepam with cathecolamine, and histamine in regions of the rat brain, in *The Ben-*

zodiazepines, Garrattini, S., Mussini, E., and Randall, L. O. (eds.), Raven Press, New York, 1973.

Teare, R. D. Some problem of barbiturate and alcoholic intoxication. *Med. Leg. J.* (Cambridge) *34*:4–10, 1966.

Teehan, B. P., Maher, J. F., Carey, J. J. H., Flynn, P. D., and Schreiner, G. E. Acute ethchlorvynol (Placidyl) intoxication. *Ann. Intern. Med. 72*:875–882, 1970.

Tengblad, K.-F. Heminevrin-enformani. *Lähartidningen 58*:1936–1942, 1961.

Teutsch, G., Mahler, D. L., Brown, C. R., Forrest, W. H., Jr., James, K. E., and Brown, B. W. Hypnotic efficacy of diphenhydremine, methapyrilene and pentobarbital. *Clin. Pharmacol. Ther. 17*:195–201, 1975.

Thompson, I. D., Dolowy, W. C., and Cole, W. H. Development of resistance of sodium pentobarbital in rats fed on a diet containing chlorcyclizine hydrochloride. *J. Pharmacol. Exp. Ther. 127*:164–166, 1959.

Thoresen, C. E., Coates, T. J., Kirmil-Gray, K., and Rosekind, M. R. Treating insomnia: A self-management approach. *Sleep Res. 7*:252, 1978.

Thoresen, C. E., Coates, T. J., Zarcone, V. P., Kirmil-Gray, K., and Rosekind, M. R. Treating the complaint of insomnia: Self-management perspectives, in *Advances in Behavioral Medicine,* Ferguson, J. M., and Taylor, C. B. (eds.), Spectrum, Englewood Cliffs, N.J., in press.

Thornby, J., Karacan, I., Searle, R., Salis, P., Ware, C., and Williams, R. Subjective reports of sleep disturbance in a Houston metropolitan health survey. Paper presented at the 17th Annual Meeting of the Association for the Psychophysiological Study of Sleep, Houston, 1977, p. 216.

Tinklenberg, J. R., Murphy, P. L., Murphy, P., Daryl, C. F., Roth, W. T., and Kopell, B. S. Drug involvement in criminal assaults by adolescents. *Arch. Gen. Psychiatry 30*:658–689, 1974.

Tokarz, T. P., and Lawrence, P. S. An analysis of temporal and stimulus factors in the treatment of insomnia. Paper presented at the Eighth Annual Meeting of the Association for the Advancement of Behavioral Therapy, Chicago, 1974.

Torry, J. M. A case of suicide with nitrazepam and alcohol. *Practitioner 217*:648–649, 1976.

Trabucchi, E., and Chiesara, E. Variezione di attivita enzimatiche e nell' effecto formace in rapport can l'eta, *G. Gerontol. Suppl. 32*:71, 1964.

Tyler, D. B. Psychological changes during experimental sleep deprivation. *Dis. Nerv. Syst. 16*:293–299, 1955.

Vajda, F., Williams, F. M., Davidson, S., Falconer, M. A., and Breckenridge, A. Human brain, cerebiospinal fluid, and plasma concentrations of diphenylhydemtoin and phenobarbital. *Clin. Pharmacol. Ther. 15*:597–603, 1974.

Velarde, N. N., and Harris, R. The effects of methyprylon on the sleep of residents of an old age home: A double-blind study. *J. Am. Geriatr. Soc. 8*:269–276, 1960.

Veldkamp, W., Straw, R. N., Metzler, C. M., and Demissianos, H. V. Efficacy and residual effect evaluation of a new hypnotic, triazolam. *J. Clin. Pharmacol. 14*:102–111, 1974.

Viukari, M., Linnoila, M., and Aalto, V. Efficacy and side affects of flurazepam, fosazepam, and nitrazepam as sleeping aids in psychogeriatric patients. *Acta Psychiatr. Scand. 57*:27–35, 1978.

Vogel, G. W. A review of REM sleep deprivation. *Arch. Gen. Psychiatry 32*:749–761, 1975.

Vogel, G. W., Traub, A. C., and Ben-Horin, P. REM deprivation. II. The effects on depressed patients. *Arch. Gen. Psychiatry 18*:301–311, 1968.

Vogel, G. W., Barker, K., Gibbons, P., and Thurmond, R. A comparison of the effects of flurazepam 30 mg and triazolam 0.5 mg on the sleep of insomniacs. *Psychopharmacology 47*:81–86, 1976.

Vogel, H. L. Intravenous use of Physostigmine in the management of acute diazepam intoxication. *J. Am. Osteopath. Assoc.* 76(5):349–351, 1977.

Wade, A., ed. *Martindale: The Extra Pharmacapoeia.* The Pharmaceutical Press, London, 1977, pp. 746–778.

Wagman, A. M. I., and Allen, R. P. Effects of alcohol ingestion and abstinence on slow wave sleep of alcoholics. *Adv. Exp. Med. Biol.* 59:453–466, 1974.

Wang, R. I. H., and Stockdale, S. L. A subjective and objective method assessing the efficacy of hypnotic medications in insomniacs, *J. Clin. Pharmacol.* 17:728–733, 1977.

Wang, I. H., Stockdale, S. L., and Hieb, E. Hypnotic efficacy of lorazepam and flurazepam. *Clin. Pharmacol. Ther.* 19(2):191–195, 1975.

Webb, W. B., and Agnew, H. W. Sleep efficiency for sleep–wake cycles of varied length. *Psychophysiology* 12:637–641, 1975.

Webb, W. B., and Friel, J. Sleep stage and personality characteristics of "natural" long and short sleepers. *Science* 171:587–588, 1971.

Weiss, H. R., Kasinoff, B. H., and Bailey, M. A. An explanation of reported sleep disturbance. *J. Nerv. Ment. Dis.* 134(6):528–534, 1962.

Weissman, M. M. The epidemiology of suicide attempts, 1960 to 1971. *Arch. Gen. Psychiatry* 30:737–746, 1974.

Weitzman, E. P., Nogeire, C., Perlow, M., Fukushima, D., Sassin, J., McGregor, P., Gallagher, T. F., and Hellman, L. Effects of prolonged 3-hour sleep–wake cycle on sleep stages, plasma cortisol, growth hormone and body temperature in man. *J. Clin. Endocrinol. Metab.* 38:1018–1030, 1974.

Welstein, L., Dement, W. C., and Mitler, M. Insomnia in the San Francisco Bay Area: A continuing survey on complaints and remedies. *Sleep Res.* 7:254, 1978. (Further data from this study is described in the Institute of Medicine, 1979, report.)

Westerfield, B. T., and Blouin, R. A. Ethchlorvynol intoxication. *South. Med. J.* 70(8), 1019–1020, 1977.

Wexler, L., Weissman, M. M., and Kasl, S. V. Suicide attempts, 1970–75: Updating a United States study and comparisons with international trends. *Br. J. Psychiatry* 132:180–185, 1978.

Whitehouse, L. W., Paul, C. J., Coldwell, B. B., and Thomas, B. H. Effect of ethanol on diazepam distribution in rat. *Res. Commun. Chem. Pathol. Pharmacol.* 12:221–242, 1975.

Whitehouse, L. W., Peterson, G., Paul, C. J., and Thomas, B. H. Effect of ethanol on the pharmacokinetics of 2-14-C-Methaqualone in the rat. *Life Sci.* 20:1871–1878, 1977.

Whitlock, F. A. The syndrome of barbiturate dependence. *Med. J. Aust.* 2:391–404, 1970.

Wiberg, G. S., Coldwell, B. B., and Trenholm, H. L. Toxicity of ethanol-barbiturate mixtures. *J. Pharm. Pharmacol.* 21:212–236, 1969.

Wiberg, G. S., Coldwell, B. B., and Trenholm, H. L. Toxicity of ethanol barbiturate mixtures. *J. Pharm. Pharmacol.* 22:465, 1970.

Wilker, A., and Rasor, R. W. Psychiatric aspects of drug addiction. *Am. J. Med.* 14:566–570, 1953.

Wilkinson, R. T. Effects of up to 60 hours' sleep deprivation on different types of work. *Ergonomics* 7:175–186, 1964.

Williams, H. L., and Salamy, A. Alcohol and sleep, in *The Biology of Alcoholism*, Kissin, B., and Begleiter, H. (eds.), Plenum Press, New York, 1972, pp. 435–483.

Williams, H. L., Lubin, A., and Goodnow, J. S. Impaired performance with acute sleep loss. *Psychol. Monogr.* 73:1–26, 1959.

Winchester, J. F., Gelfand, M. C., Knepshield, J. H., and Schreiner, G. E. Dialysis and hemoperfusion of poisons and drugs—update. *Trans. Am. Soc. Artif. Intern. Organs* 23:762–842, 1977.

Winfield, D. L., and Hughes, J. G. The use of noludar in pediatric electroencephalography. *Electroencephalogr. Clin. Neurophysiol. 9*:713–715, 1957.

Winne, D. Die Bedeutung der Blutdränope in der Pharmacokinetik der entiralen Resorption. *Med. Welt 16*:632, 1971.

Wise, C. D., Berger, B. D., and Stein, L. Benzodiazepines: Anxiety-reducing activity by reduction of serotonin turnover in the brain. *Science 177*:180–183, 1972.

Wissler, E. Pathogenese und Prognose der Hypnoticaabhängigkeit. *Schweiz. Arch. Neurol. Neurochir. Psychiatr. 104*:389–425, 1969.

Wolff, B. B. Evaluation of hypnotics in outpatients with insomnia using a questionnaire and a self-rating technique. *Clin. Pharmacol. Ther. 15*(2):130–140, 1974.

World Health Organization. WHO expert committee on drug dependence. Technical Report Series No. 407, 1969, pp. 1–28.

World Health Organization. Report of a WHO Scientific Group: Evaluation of dependence liability and dependence potential of drugs. Technical Report Series 577, 1975, pp. 1–50.

Wyatt, R. J. The serotonin–catecholamine dream bicycle: A clinical study. *Biol. Psychiatry 5*:33–63, 1972.

Yanagita, T., and Takahashi, S. Development of tolerance to and physical dependence on barbiturates in rhesus monkey. *J. Pharmacol. Exp. Therap. 172*:163–169, 1970.

Young, R. E., Ramsay, L. E., and Murray, T. S. Barbiturates and serum calcium in the elderly. *Postgrad. Med. J. 53*:212–215, 1977.

Yules, R. B., Lippman, M. E., and Freedman, D. X. Alcohol administration prior to sleep: The effect on EEG sleep stages. *Arch. Gen. Psychiatry 16*:94–97, 1967.

Zbinden, G., and Randall, L. O. Pharmacology of benzodiazepines: Laboratory and clinical correlations. *Adv. Pharmacol. 5*:213–291, 1967.

Zilly, W. Arzneimittelelimination (Hexabarbital, Tolbutamid Digoxin and B-Methyldigoxin) bei Patienten mit akuter Hepatitis und Leberzirrhose. M.D. thesis, Univ. of Wurzburg, Fed. Rep. of German, 1974.

Zilly, W., Brachtel, D., and Richter, E. Hexobarbital-Plasmapiegel Patienten mit akuter Hepatitis während kontinuierlicher Hexobarbital-Infusion. *Klin. Wochenschr. 51*:346–347, 1973.

Zimmerman, W. B. Psychological and physiological differences between "light" and "deep" sleepers. Unpublished doctoral dissertation, University of Chicago, 1967.

Zorick, F., Roth, T., Salio, P., Kramer, M., and Lutz, T. Insomnia and excessive daytime sleepiness as presenting symptoms in nocturnal myoclonus. *Sleep Res. 7*:256, 1978.

Zung, W. W. K. The effect of placebo and drugs on human sleep. *Biol. Psychiatry 6*:89–92, 1973.

Index

Abuse
  hypnotic, 128
Acetylcholine, 10–13
Advertising
  over-the-counter hypnotics, 153
Alcohol
  associated with insomnia, 20
  interaction with hypnotics, 115–125
  as treatment of insomnia, 160–161
Amobarbital. *See* Barbiturates
D-Amphetamine, 10
Amylobarbitone. *See* Barbiturates
Antipyrine, 143
Apomorphine, 97

Barbiturates
  actions of, 47
  alcohol and, 166–168
  altered metabolism in the elderly, 50–52
  chronic administration of, 51–52
  crime and, 129
  dependence on, 128–138
  efficacy of, 70–72
  in elderly, 142–152
  history of, 45–46
  residual effects of, 102–111
  structure and classification of, 42–50
  suicides and, 90, 92
  toxicity, 92–93
Benzodiazepines
  dependence, 136
  history, 52–53

Benzodiazepines (*cont.*)
  interaction with alcohol, 118–122
  overdose, 93
  residual effects, 108
  See also Flurazepam; Nitrazepam;
    Temazepam
Berger, Hans, 1
Biofeedback, 166–169
Bromides, 156
Butabarbital. *See* Barbiturates

Caton, Richard, 1
Charcoal
  activated, 97
Chloral hydrate
  efficacy, 78–79
  in elderly, 148–149
  interaction with alcohol, 122–123
  overdoses, 93–94
  pharmacology, 56–58
Chlordiazepoxide. *See* Benzodiazepines
Clonidine, 10
Cocaine, 10
Conditioning
  classical, 170–171
Consciousness
  states of, 3
Control
  stimulus, 170–171
Counseling, 163–164
Cycle, Basic Rest Activity (BRAC), 6
Cycle, REM–nonREM, 6

Delta sleep, 5
Density, REM, 6
Dependence
    hypnotic, 127–139
Depression
    associated with insomnia, 20
    hypnotics in, 68–69
    suicide and, 90
Desensitization
    systematic, 169–170
Diazepam
    dependence, 134, 136
    and driving, 112
    interaction with alcohol, 118–121
    psychomotor effects, 105
Dichloralphenazone. See Chloral hydrate
Digit–Symbol Substitution Test (DSST)
    description, 104
    effects of hypnotics on, 104–105
Diphenhydramine, 155, 158
Disorders of initiating and maintaining
        sleep (DIMS), 20–22
Distribution
    volume of, 44
L-Dopa, 10
Dopamine, 10
Doxylamine, 158
Dreaming, 2–3
Driving, 112

Efficacy
    hypnotic, 63–84
Elderly
    efficacy of hypnotics in, 145–150
    pharmacology in, 142–144
    toxicity of hypnotics in, 150–151
    use of hypnotics, 28, 141
Electroencephalogram (EEG), 1, 3
Emesis, 97
Ethchlorvynol
    dependence, 128
    efficacy, 83
    overdose, 94–95
    pharmacology, 60
Ethinamate
    dependence, 128
    pharmacology, 61
    toxicity, 94
Excedrin-PM®, 148–149, 157
Eysenck, H. J., 164

Field. See Gigantocellular tegmental field
Flurazepam
    dependence, 128
    efficacy, 72–76
    in elderly, 146–147
    interaction with alcohol, 120–121
    overdoses, 93
    pharmacology, 53–55
    residual effects, 102–112
Food and Drug Administration, 157–159

Gamma aminobutyric acid (GABA), 13
Gigantocellular tegmental field (FTG),
        10–11
Glutethimide
    dependence, 128
    efficacy, 81
    in elderly, 148–149
    interaction with alcohol, 123–124
    overdose, 94–95
    pharmacology, 59–60
    residual effects, 106–107, 110

Half-life, 44
Hemodialysis, 97–98
Hemoperfusion, 98
Hexobarbital. See Barbiturates
Humors
    circulating, 12
Hypnotics
    alcohol and, 115–125
    dependence on, 127–139
    EEG effects, 101–103
    efficacy of, 63–83
    elderly and, 141–151
    frequency of use, 31–34
    number of prescriptions for
        inpatients, 36–37
        outpatients, 35–36
    pharmacology of
        nonprescription, 153–156
        prescription, 39–61
    physicians who prescribe, 35
    regulation of, 157–159
    residual effects of, 101–113
    suicide and, 85–99
    treatment of toxicity, 96–98
Hypnotoxin. See Sleep regulation,
        circulating humors
Hyptor®, 148

Insomnia
    alternative pharmacologic treatments
        for, 153–161
    approach to the patient with, 182–185
    childhood, 22
    conditions associated with, 19–22
    description, 16
    experience of, 18
    and length of sleep, 17
    nonpharmacologic treatment of,
        163–175
    prevalence, 25–30
    types of complaints, 31
Intubation, 97

Jet lag, 22, 68

K complex, 4

Latency
    REM, 6
    sleep, 6
Locus coeruleus, 10

Mandrax®. See Methaqualone
Methapyriline, 154–155
Methaqualone
    efficacy, 79–81
    in elderly, 148–149
    interaction with alcohol, 123
    overdose, 84
    pharmacology, 58–59
    residual effects, 106–107, 110
Methylphenidate, 10
Methyprylon
    dependence, 128
    efficacy, 82
    overdose, 94
    pharmacology, 60
Methysergide, 10
Minnesota Multiphasic Personality
        Inventory (MMPI), 20, 164–165
Myoclonus
    nocturnal
        associated with insomnia, 21
        hypnotics in patients with, 68

Neurotransmitters, 10–12
Nitrazepam
    dependence, 131
    efficacy, 76–77

Nitrazepam (cont.)
    in elderly, 146–147
    overdoses, 93
    pharmacology, 55
    residual effects, 102–103, 106–107
    withdrawal, 77, 138
Nonprescription hypnotics. See
        Over-the-counter hypnotics
NonREM sleep, 4–5
Norepinephrine, 10

Over-the-counter hypnotics
    contents, 154–156
    efficacy of, 156–157
    quantities used, 153–154
    regulation of, 157–159

Parachlorophenylalanine (PCPA), 10, 159
Pentobarbital
    efficacy, 70–72
    pharmacology, 49
    See also Barbiturates
Performance
    daytime, 104–111
Pharmacology, general
    absorption, 41
    alterations in the elderly, 142–144
    biotransformation, 142–144
    excretion, 44
    protein binding, 41–42
    solubility, 40–41
    volume of distribution, 44
Phase lag, 9, 22
Phenobarbital. See Barbiturates
Phenyltoloxamine, 158
Physostigmine, 11, 96
Pimozide, 11
Pontine-geniculate-occipital spikes
        (PGO), 10–11
Prescribing
    recommendations for, 184–185
Psychotherapy, 163–164

Raphe nuclei, 10
Reaction time
    description, 106
    effects of hypnotics on, 106–107
Regulation, Federal, 157–159
Relaxation
    progressive, 166–169
    See also Biofeedback

REM sleep
  in alcoholism, 160
  description, 6
  in hypnotic withdrawal, 14, 72, 75, 138
  regulation of, 10–11
Restless legs syndrome, 21
Rhythm
  alpha, 3, 166
  beta, 3
  delta, 5
  theta, 4, 166

Scopolamine, 11, 155–156
Secobarbital
  pharmacology, 49
  See also Barbiturates
Self-management
  behavioral, 173–174
Serotonin, 10
Sleep Apnea
  associated with insomnia, 20–21
  hypnotics in patients with, 67
Sleep
  deprivation, 12–15
  latency, 6
  need for, 15–16
  regulation
    circulating humors, 12
    hypnotics and, 12–13
    passive versus active model, 9–10
    role of neurotransmitters, 10–12
  spindles, 4
  stages
    descriptions of, 3–7
    influences on appearance of
      age, 7–8
      circadian effects, 7–9
      duration of prior wakefulness, 7
      duration of sleep, 7
Sleepers
  good and poor, 18
  light and deep, 17
  natural short and long, 16
Sleeping pills. See Hypnotics
Slow-wave sleep
  in alcoholism, 160
  description, 5
  effects of flurazepam on, 75–76

Solubility
  hypnotic, 40–41
Spikes. See Pontine-geniculate- occipital
    spikes
Steady state, 44–45
Stearnbach, Leo, 52
Suicide
  incidence, 85–89
  prevention, 98
  victims of, 89–92
System
  reticular activating, 9

Tapping rate
  description, 106
  effects of hypnotics on, 106–107
Temazepam
  efficacy, 77–78
  pharmacology, 55
Temperature
  body, 165
Tests
  psychomotor, 104–105, 108–111
Thalidomide, 94
Therapy
  attributional, 171–172
  behavioral, 164–175
Toxicity
  hypnotic
    acute, 92–96
    in elderly, 150–151
Tracking test
  description, 104
  effects of hypnotics on, 106–107
Training
  autogenic, 166–169
Triazolam
  efficacy, 72, 74
  in elderly, 146–147
  residual effects, 102–103, 106–107
  withdrawal, 138
Triclofos. See Chloral hydrate
Tripp, Peter, 13
L-Tryptophan, 159

vonBaeyer, Adolph, 45–46